Pathways of Hope

Living Well with Cognitive Changes

*A bond exists between all things
because they all drink the same water
and breathe the same air.*

—LUTHER STANDING BEAR,
LAKOTA CHIEF OF THE OGLALA

edited by Christine Baum Van Ryzin,
Mary Kay Baum,
and Rosann Baum Milius
on behalf of *forMemory*, Inc.

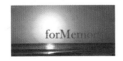

Elemental Basic Publishing
Appleton, Wisconsin

Registered with the Library of Congress
ISBN: 978-0-9761336-3-6

Published by Elemental Basic Publishing
P.O. Box 571, Appleton, WI 54912
www.elementalbasicpub.com

This book was published with the help of the Alzheimer's & Dementia Alliance of Wisconsin (ADAW), who provide advocacy, library, newsletter and support groups for individuals living with Alzheimer's and related diseases. Contact them at 517 N. Segoe Rd., Madison, WI 53705; 608-232-3400; toll-free at 888-308-6251; email support@alzwisc.org; or **www.alzwisc.org**, with offices also in Lancaster and Portage.

In part *forMemory* is supported by a "Building Bridges of Hope in Early Onset Dementia" grant from Wheat Ridge Ministries, seeding health and hope (**www.wheatridge.org**).

We also thank the South-Central Synod of Wisconsin, ELCA.

Design and layout were donated by Jane Rundell of Mazomanie, Wisc.

Most photography is by Mary Kay Baum of Dodgeville, Wisc. and is donated. She was assisted by The Camera Company and Meuer Art and Picture Frame Co., both of Madison, Wisc.

Printing was done by Park Printing of Verona, Wisc.

A suggested donation of $18 helps printing and distribution.
We urge larger tax-deductible contributions to provide books in volume to Alzheimer chapters, support groups, clergy, libraries, medical personnel, clinics, and affected families.

To participate, see **www.formemory.org**. To mail a tax-deductible donation, send a check made out to *forMemory, Inc.* to Rosann Milius, 1305 Maricopa Drive, Oshkosh, WI 54904. Contact 1-920-231-9237, rosann.milius@gmail.com. To make a credit card donation, volunteer, ask for a speaker, or order more copies of *Pathways of Hope*, call Chris Van Ryzin at 1-920-734-9638.

Contents

Learn from yesterday, live for today, hope for tomorrow.
The important thing is to not stop questioning.

—ALBERT EINSTEIN

Foreword

Craig S. Atwood, Ph.D.

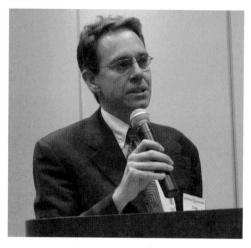

This short book with its inviting photographs, inspiring stories and beautiful layout embodies the efforts of a group of individuals involved in an important revolutionary movement. This movement is made up of persons who, while diagnosed early in life (typically in their 40's and 50's) with a disease that leads to dementia, are taking action. Its contributors describe their lives with memory challenges; their relationships and support of those similarly affected; their combined use of Western and Eastern medicines; their fight for recognition of their plight; and their fight for memory. As you will read, they write with passion and care for our common futures, linking human health and world wellness. They are *forMemory*, and this is their story.

Alzheimer's disease afflicts around 5.3 million individuals and is the sixth leading cause of death in the US [Alzheimer's Association, 2010; Centers for Disease Control and Prevention (CDC) National Center for Health Statistics]. Its toll on our community is measured in terms of both the emotional burden it places on families and friends, as well as the large number of unpaid caregivers (10.9 million) and annual cost of this disease to our society ($172 billion). African-Americans and Hispanics are at higher risk

for developing Alzheimer's disease, being ~2 times and 1.5 times more likely than Caucasians to develop the disease, respectively.

The Wisconsin Alzheimer's Institute estimates that one in three families in Wisconsin are now affected by dementia and having a mother with Alzheimer's disease puts one at significantly greater risk than having a father with Alzheimer's disease. Females themselves experience a higher prevalence of Alzheimer's disease than males. Statistics tell us that a baby girl born in Wisconsin today has a life expectancy of one hundred years. Statistics also tell us that one half of these girls will develop dementia in their lifetimes unless we make major changes to the system designed to provide therapies; unless we prevent or at least treat individuals before the onset of cognitive damage.

It is estimated that early onset forms of Alzheimer's disease (before 65 years of age) account for 2–5% of those who succumb to the disease. This equates to 105,000–265,000 individuals with this early, chronic and progressive form of the disease that impacts normal function at an age when most are in their prime. These individuals live with the disease from the time they are cognizant of the effects of the disease on their parents and grandparents, through to the development of the disease in themselves and finally through their children and grandchildren. *forMemory* is comprised of a group of such middle-aged individuals who have taken it upon themselves to experiment at both the social and medical levels in an attempt to halt the onset of the disease, lessen the effects of this disease and to slow the progression of the disease. In essence, to find a solution where traditional medicine and research endeavors have failed.

To understand a disease, you must study the disease. The members of *forMemory* have in effect performed a large scientific experiment, testing tens if not hundreds of different medicines and combinations of medicines and other therapies on themselves in efforts to find a solution to a disease that they live with, and must cope with, every day of their lives. This book is a compilation of many stories of their attempts to offset this disease, and their search for hope.

forMemory has taken it upon themselves to develop and compile these anecdotal case reports into a database that will eventually be available online for all to access. These anecdotal results will be a veritable treasure chest of first hand experiences to guide basic and social scientists. It is hope for those with family histories of dementia diseases. It is hope for all families with dementia. It is also a motivator for the general public and for policy makers to effect systemic changes in the way diseases are researched.

Alzheimer's disease is the result of a combination of genetic and environmental factors that leads to progressive sub-clinical neurodegeneration over many years that finally manifests as cognitive impairment. My own research that examines how hormonal changes with aging lead to neurodegenerative diseases has been informed by the work of *forMemory* and other anecdotal cases, and vice versa, and is an important demonstration of how anecdotal reports can inform future research directions.

Interventions are required at every point on the neurodegenerative cascade in order to halt this disease. An important intervention involves physiological (bio-identical to human) hormone replacement therapy (HRT). While HRT has been inappropriately maligned, it is to date the only therapy to be proven, in eight clinical trials, to not only halt the progression of the disease, but to actually enhance cognition in those with Alzheimer's disease. Another intervention found helpful by some with cognitive problems has been the prescription drug selegiline. Developed primarily for Parkinson's disease and for depression, it illustrates the heterogeneous nature of dementia.

Nonprescription interventions are also found to be important. Adults who exercise their brains are two and a half times less likely to develop Alzheimer's disease. So Sudoku, for example, is an intellectually stimulating game that may slow the age-related loss of hard wiring that we all experience. And there is now virtually universal consensus that exercise is a significant intervention and helps maintain brain health. The personal accounts in this book relay how individuals have incorporated strategies such as these into their own lives.

I first became informed of *forMemory* while being interviewed by Mona Johnson for her website The Tangled Neuron. I subsequently was introduced to Chris Baum Van Ryzin and Mary Kay Baum from which the seeds of the current endeavor began to sprout, as it became evident that not only the early members of *forMemory*, but tremendous numbers of other similarly afflicted individuals, were exploring various therapies. I have enjoyed collaborating with *forMemory* on its database project. The courage and wisdom of these individuals to move beyond the bounds of the current system to find solutions must be applauded, especially as they try to raise awareness of these solutions. Their efforts have been appreciated by those experiencing early-onset memory challenges, laypersons and scientists alike through their presentations at meetings such as the annual Wisconsin State Alzheimer's conference and the 2008 International Conference on Alzheimer's disease.

I congratulate *forMemory* not only for their proactive stance in fighting this disease, but for their forward-thinking efforts to involve youth and provide respite activities for teens of affected families. Together may we open pathways of hope toward preventing dementias in current and future generations.

Craig S. Atwood received his Ph.D. from the University of Western Australia, Perth. He has held various faculty positions at Harvard Medical School, Case Western Reserve University and the University of Wisconsin-Madison where he is currently an Associate Professor in the Department of Medicine.

He is Research Director of the Wisconsin Alzheimer's Institute and of the Wisconsin Comprehensive Memory Program; a Health Science Specialist in the Geriatric Research, Education and Clinical Center at the William S. Middleton Memorial Veterans Administration Hospital, Madison, Wisc.; an Adjunct Professor in the Department of Pathology, Case Western Reserve University, Cleveland, Ohio; and an Adjunct Senior Lecturer, Edith Cowan University, School of Biomedical & Sports Science, Faculty of Computing, Health and Science, Perth, West Australia; Head of the Laboratory of Endocrinology, Aging and Disease (LEAD).

Dr. Atwood has authored more than 120 peer-reviewed research and review articles, has a h-index = 38 and is a member of numerous editorial boards including the *Journal of Alzheimer's Disease, Current Alzheimer's Research, Journal of Biological Chemistry, Neural Regeneration Research, Nutrition and Diabetes*, and the *International Journal of Clinical and Experimental Medicine*. In 2004 Dr. Atwood co-authored a major new theory of aging, "The Reproductive Cell-Cycle Theory of Aging," that explains why and how we age at the evolutionary, physiological and molecular levels. He regularly presents seminars to the larger community on aging, aging-related diseases such as Alzheimer's disease, and strategies to halt the aging process. He is a recipient of the Zenith Fellow Award from the Alzheimer's Association.

Selected Publications

Atwood C.S. and Bowen R.L. (2011). The reproductive-cell cycle theory of aging: An update. *Experimental Gerontology*. 2010 Sep 17. [Epub ahead of print]

Atwood, C.S. and Vadakkadath Meethal, S. (2011). Gonadotropins and Progestogens: Obligatory Developmental Functions during Early Embryogenesis and their Role in Adult Neurogenesis, Neuroregeneration, and Neurodegeneration. In: *Hormones in Neurodegeneration, Neuroprotection and Neurogenesis*, Eds. Achille Gravanis and Synthia Mellon, Wiley-Blackwell (in press).

Bowen, R.L. and Atwood, C.S. (2004). Living and Dying for Sex: A theory of aging based on the modulation of cell cycle signaling by reproductive hormones. *Gerontology*, 50(5), 265–290.

Bowen, R.L., Verdile, G., Liu, T., Perry, G., Smith, M.A., Martins, R.N. and Atwood, C.S. (2004). Luteinizing hormone, a reproductive regulator that modulates the processing of amyloid-ß protein precursor and amyloid-ß deposition. *Journal of Biological Chemistry*, 279(19), 20539–45.

Gallego, M.J., Porayette, P., Kaltcheva, M.M., Bowen, R.L., Vadakkadath Meethal, S. and Atwood, C. S. (2010). The pregnancy hormones human chorionic gonadotropin and progesterone induce human embryonic stem cell proliferation and differentiation into neuroectodermal rosettes. *Stem Cell Research & Therapy*, 1:28.

Haasl, R.J., Reza Ahmadi, M., Vadakkadath Meethal, S., Gleason, C.E., Johnson, S.C., Asthana, S., Bowen, R.L. and Atwood, C.S. (2008). A luteinizing hormone receptor intronic variant is significantly associated with decreased risk of Alzheimer's disease in males carrying an apolipoprotein E ε4 Allele. *BMC Medical Genetics*, 9(1):37.

Liu, T., Wimalasena, J., Bowen, R.L. and Atwood, C.S. (2007). Luteinizing hormone receptor mediates neuronal pregnenolone production via upregulation of steroidogenic acute regulatory protein expression. *Journal of Neurochemistry*, 100(5), 1329–1339.

Porayette, P., Gallego, M.J., Kaltcheva, M.M., Bowen, R.L., Vadakkadath Meethal, S. and Atwood, C.S. (2009). Differential processing of amyloid-beta precursor protein directs human embryonic stem cell proliferation and differentiation into neuronal precursor cells. *Journal of Biological Chemistry*, 284(35), 23806–23817.

Wilson, A.C., Clemente, L., Liu, T., Bowen, R.L., Vadakkadath Meethal, S. and Atwood, C.S. (2008). Reproductive hormones regulate the selective permeability of the blood-brain barrier. *Biochimica et Biophysica Acta – Molecular Basis of Disease*, 1782(6), 401–407.

I. Introduction in Verse

Learning to love is why we are here on earth. It means expanding our circle
of care and compassion beyond our family and friends to all living beings,
to all of creation. Learning to love is a long and winding pathway
and the source of all meaning on this earth.

(paraphrase of Vincent Kavaloski in *Living the Questions:
Philosophy as the Search for Meaning and Mystery*)

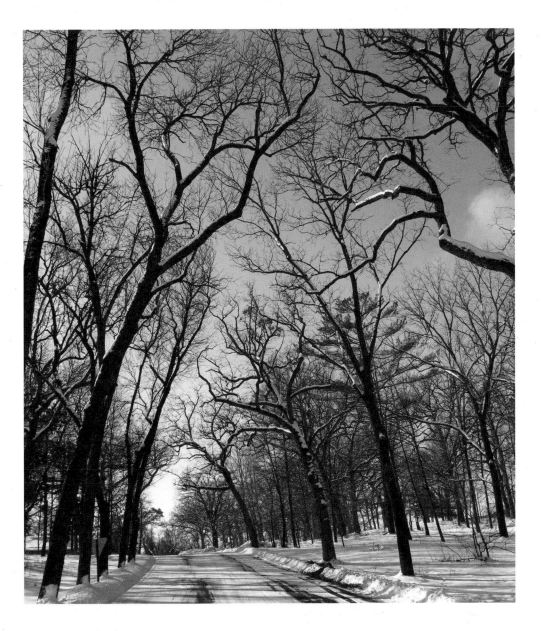

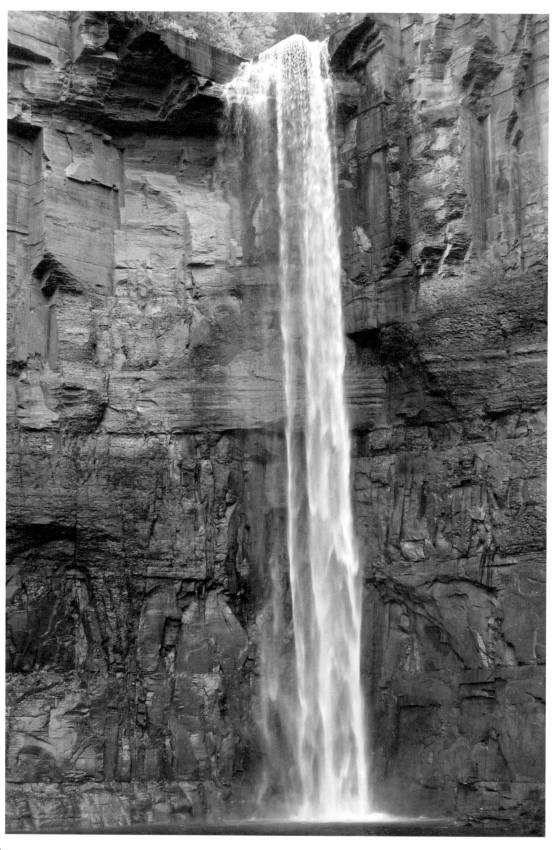

Ever wonder why I don't like to take a bath or shower?

It is time for my shower. But before I start I go to my husband and tell him I am going to take a shower.

I never did that before, why now?

I am in the shower. There are so many things to remember:

Controlling the water—which way is hot? How do I make it cooler?
How do I keep the water from drowning me?

And all that water, hitting me . . . like a thousand questions attacking my body . . . over and over. Distracting. Too fast for my sense of touch! Too fast for my brain!

Soap
Wash cloth
Wet my hair
Shampoo
Rinse

And all that water, hitting me . . . like a thousand questions attacking my body . . . over and over. Distracting. Too fast for my sense of touch! Too fast for my brain!

Did I shampoo?
Did I cream rinse?
Do I need to rinse?

And all that water, hitting me . . . like a thousand questions attacking my body . . . over and over. Distracting. Too fast for my sense of touch! Too fast for my brain!

Don't hold the razor so hard—it will cut.
Don't fall.
Am I safe?

And all that water, hitting me . . . like a thousand questions attacking my body . . . over and over. Distracting. Too fast for my sense of touch! Too fast for my brain!

I could not understand why it was getting harder and harder to take a shower or bath. Until one day when I was in the shower and the phone rang. I reached for the portable phone. It was my daughter. I was so exhausted from a simple shower that used to be refreshing—but no longer. I asked her if she ever realized how many parts there are to a simple shower and just how hard it can really be to remember each one?

And all that water, hitting me . . . like a thousand questions attacking my body . . . over and over. Distracting. Too fast for my sense of touch! Too fast for my brain!

There came a day, not so very long ago, when I was standing in the shower and was no longer frightened by the water hitting my face! In an instant, I fully understood what had been happening to me. What a great feeling—to once again actually enjoy the feel of water!

No more overload . . .

From a talk given by Christine Baum Van Ryzin: "Learn to Listen with Your Heart: Insights into Alzheimer's Disease from a Person Challenged by Early Onset Alzheimer's Disease"

New Openings, New Pathways

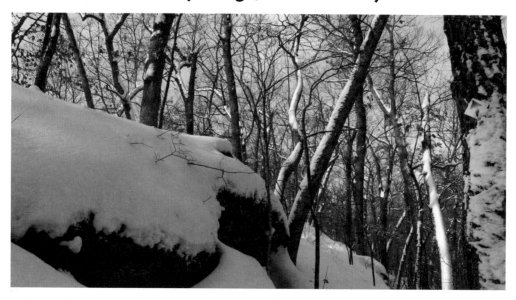

Our mothers waited for new ways.
Our mothers had to live their fears alone.
Our aunts cried their laments alone,
They were angry that words had left them.
Cousins were isolated, not knowing what the other was going through.

Now a new thing is happening.
We meet others like ourselves, we see similarities.
We are not, after all, alone in how we've changed
We see many others like us.

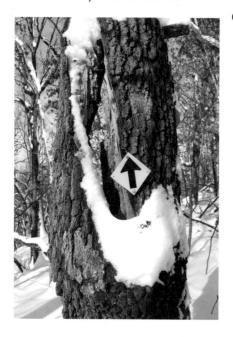

Others are also feeling overloaded,
  and skipping favorite activities,
  becoming more clumsy,
  knocking into things,
  being slower at everything,
  feeling the weight of fatigue,

  distracted by commotion,
  easily overwhelmed,
  losing our train of thought,
  not finding our words,

  losing track of time,
  losing keys, cell phone and calendar,
  arriving late or not at all,

  not sleeping so well,
  not letting go of our troubles,

  having to take careful notes,
  but misplacing the notes,

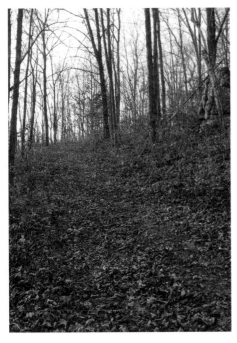

offended by teasing,
hearing it as criticism,
feeling attacked by questions,

feeling queasy about many cleaners,
getting headaches from some foods,
getting dizzy from chlorine water,
feeling weak from polluted air and water,

being afraid in once familiar places.

Sometimes we feel "on,"
    unpredictably we feel in a daze.
We feel exhausted by writing this much.

We take notice of these little changes,
    so subtle, but so real.

We are workers who were let go,
    or were fired, or demoted,
    or we retired early.
We couldn't take it anymore.

Our mothers died of something called Alzheimer's.
So did some aunts.
Besides acting confused,
    we found them cranky, distracted,
    we thought they didn't like us any more.
We feared we'd be like that.

But now there is hope.
We can speak and we listen to one another
We share ways we learned to live with
    changes.
We are test pilots for remedies and
    research.
We reveal what works well for us.
The more we listen, the more we learn
    about ourselves.
We discover new pathways and wise old
    trails.
Our mothers still inspire us.
Our daughters start to hear our stories.
Our neighbors take notice.

The earth applauds our wisdom
    for seeing links to environment.
The trees sing out with us.
We marked our favorite trails, the pathways
    that opened new directions for us.
Together we find our words, our voices.

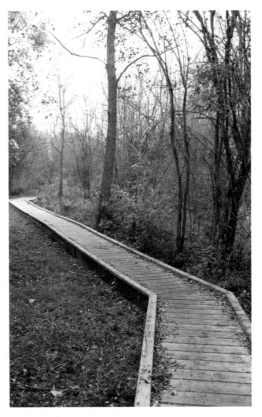

We are the ones who can say what it's like.
We can tell what helps,
    what hurts,
    and what we want.

We can mark paths we've explored,
    lanes to follow and hazards to avoid.

If someday we do become mute,
    the stones will still stand in for us,
    marking the healing places
    for our children's children.

Our mothers had been waiting for us.
Our aunts had been hoping for us.

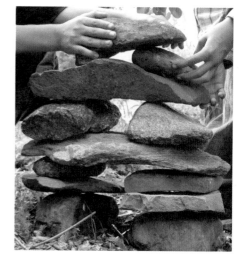

—*Rev. Mary Kay Baum*

Inspired by Hebrew Scriptures of Jeremiah 30–31, Joel 2:28, and Habakkuk 2:11, and by Newer Testament counterparts Acts 2:17 and Luke 19:40: "I tell you, if these do become silent, even the very stones will cry out."

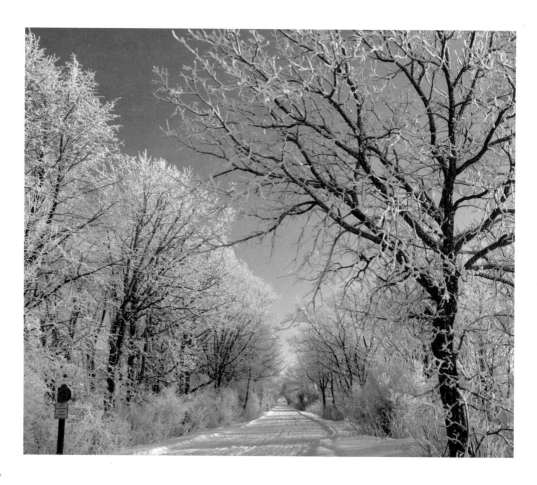

Relearning to Learn is Relearning to Live

With a diagnosis we go through
    Fear
    Anger
    Grief
    Depression.
We meet others and find
    Hope that the brain is repairable
    Reasons to keep on living
    Places to start in our strengths
    Encouragement to speak out.
We choose our personal goals and
    Act pacing one step at a time
    Considering it fun, creative, and an
      adventure.
We evaluate and change directions or
simplify
    Maybe several times a day.

We address fatigue by resting and
    Restarting again later.
We accept surprising outcomes with
satisfaction.
We know process is more important
than expectations.
We affirm ourselves for our efforts.
We understand that another attempt
later might be easier.
We are gaining wisdom to balance
    Enough mental and creative activity
    Enough social connection and
      exercise
    Enough medication and nutrition
    Enough sleep, rest, and appreciation
      of life.

—*Christine Baum Van Ryzin*

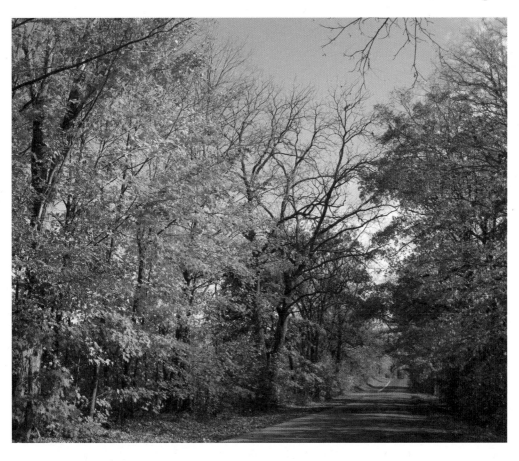

The Path

I give shape to the farm
Connecting all that it holds.
Edged by fences,
Rutted by tractor tires and hooves,
Finely tuned by bicycle tires spun and
    swirled,
I am the lane.

Open my gate that forms the beginning
Endless to little eyes.
Parts are dry sand with a rocky edge,
Others soft with moss in the shade
    of a tree.
A roller coaster of uneven land
Ever changing yet the same.
Feel secure in my form.

Experience the fields as they pass by.
Look close as you choose your way.

I am wide enough for change.
Some footprints follow the paths
    of others,
Others venture to higher ground.
Each forms my uniqueness
As long as you take the next step.

Rest under a tree
Buzzing with life as bees nest in its
    womb.
See where you have been.
By coming you have left a change in
    me.
Simple at the end I blend into a vast
    field.
Journey on . . .
I am your life

—*Christine Baum Van Ryzin*

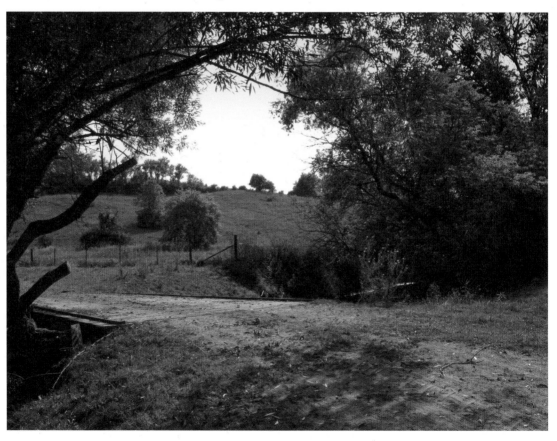

II. Individuals Tell Their Stories

"We want our lives to be about life. We want to be with people who are working on life, and build connections that help us help each other do that year after year until we hand our work over to others. We want to hear songs . . . We want to make the choices and take the risks that make possible the next generation."

—Gary Gunderson in *Leading Causes of Life*

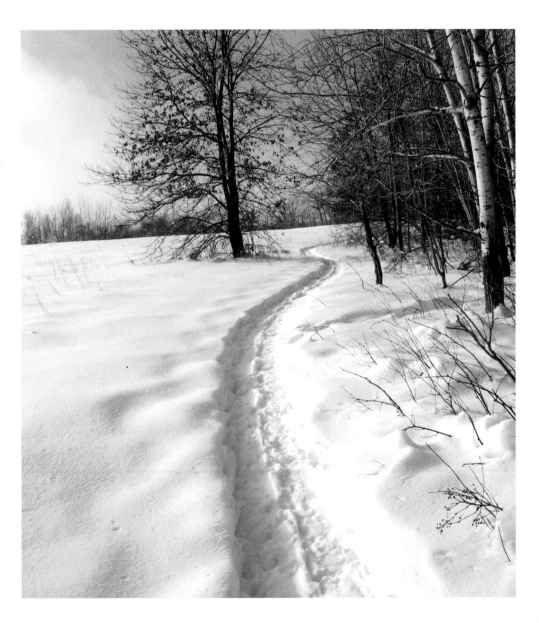

I Continue to Seek Answers

Chris Baum Van Ryzin

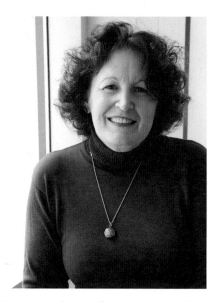

I was 41 when I first experienced symptoms like those we'd seen in our mother in her fifties. By then she was 70. My symptoms included memory problems, tremors, weakness especially in arms and legs, personality changes—quickened temper, and a stiff face with a forced smile. That was in 1989, before early onset was acknowledged. I was in limbo for more than 10 years. During that time I told my family that my face was not expressing my feelings. If I looked mad, I probably was not. So remember, I would still be smiling on the inside. Not until our mother's death and autopsy in 1995 —as well as my older sister's symptoms, which appeared in 1999—did we have a clearer diagnosis. Those were terrible years because I felt every loss and knew my only hope was early detection. And I wasn't getting it!

Hope came in 1995 when studies showed that the brain was repairable, a gift of life. My journey would not have to follow our mother's. I slipped away into a world focused on finding the "how." This focus was often seen as an obsession, but it was what I

had to do for myself, my family and children. By 1998, I could no longer remember what I should know. I couldn't cook, I didn't know which clothes I owned so every day was a struggle to dress. I was weak, unable to tolerate heat or cold, and I couldn't get the words out. I had developed and managed with my family Galaxy Science and Hobby Center, an Appleton retail store and center for learning and discovery. I was no longer able to work with the customers, not remembering the answers to their questions. I was often seen as gruff and unfriendly—so not me. Dr. Benjamin Brooks, neurologist and researcher wrote, ". . . looking older than her stated age with a sad grimace on her face." My husband hung onto me, filling my days with healing endorphins. "Laughter is the best medicine." Even if he hardly received an outward response from me.

The turning point came when our grandson was born in 1999. I was put onto a plane in Wisconsin and was picked up at the airport by my son-in-law in Washington DC. Max was just a day old. I was so excited to meet our first grandchild and found I had a new identity, a grandmother. But even more happened—during the month there I watched him struggle to learn, trying over and over. I realized that if I was going to become "like a child" in this disease, then maybe if I took the energy I was using in trying to maintain and instead restarted as a child to relearn and move forward instead of backward it might work. I decided to follow my grandson's example: one hour of learning stimulation, one hour of nutrition, and one hour of rest/sleep. As I nurtured my grandson, I was able to relearn how to nurture myself in a whole mind, body, and spirit approach. And the regimen started to work!

I accepted my losses, an emotional step that helped clear negative attitudes. Before I could move forward I needed to know what

I could or couldn't do. I recognized my limitations and how to work with them. Even now, I function more slowly and do my best thinking in a quiet place. I recognized my need to take breaks and de-stress, usually through right-brain activities like writing and designing. "Do less now, so you can do more later."

At a May 2000 neurology appointment we discussed our new grandson and what I was learning. Dr. Brooks stated, "You don't look like a grandmother!" The approach of nurturing the whole mind, body, and spirit was making a difference.

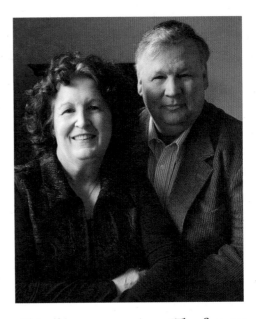

Brain injury, inflammation, oxidation, nutrition, were to become key words. Taking all that researchers were working on, my family and I began to combine an Eastern and Western approach to manage the disease. Working with Dr. Brooks and others on my team, over the years I included herbs, topical anti-inflammatory lotions and nutritional supplements to enhance the medications. I reduced inflammation with a soaking herb bath. I reduced stress by finding my place of bliss, doing light meditation, and humming. I eliminated toxic food additives including monosodium glutamate and aspartame. I chose organic foods and avoided environmental toxins, even bringing my own bedding to hotels to avoid my reaction to their bleach and fabric softener. I learned the importance of both physical and mental exercise.

By 2003 I considered myself a survivor—not cured, but no longer in decline! I took all my accumulated research and started to organize it for my family. I ended up self-publishing a book in 2004, *Alzheimer's Averted: A Path to Survival.* I published the second edition in 2009, available in soft cover for $18 at www.alzheimersaverted.com or at our family business, Galaxy Science and Hobby Center, Appleton, Wisconsin, 920-730-9220.

I never expected what happened next—that each year I would continue to get a little better. The puzzle pieces continue to come together even now. My husband likes to break it into being married to three wives within the same marriage. "The first one took a lot of good chances," Wade states of our first 20 years of marriage. Our mother always told us to never feel bad for trying something and failing, only feel bad if we didn't take the chance to try, so I often looked outside the box. The second was with the out-of-control years down the path of cognitive decline. "It was a dark time, kind of like 'The Lord of the Rings'," he states. "I never knew what was happening or what was going to happen when I walked through the door from work." The third is calmer, the living with and challenged by limitations. Fear has been replaced with knowledge. My husband now reports that my flirty smile is coming more easily, and that our world, which had grown quiet, is now frequently filled with chatty conversation. Together we share new values in life. We are OK as we celebrate our 42nd wedding anniversary. "I am proud of you for the help and hope you bring to so many people." he states as we come home from a conference.

In healing I have added the knowledge of one being cared for to my knowledge of care partner. I share this knowledge freely. Ever wonder why I . . . ? Ever wonder if I . . . ? My questions continue to be answered through the years. It was at a conference not long ago that I understood why it was

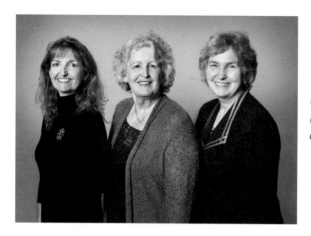

The three sisters, Rosann Milius, Chris Van Ryzin, and Mary Kay Baum at a 2011 family event.

painful when I was touched—even in a loving way. A hug hurt—I was careful not to flinch when my husband reached out with a hug or touch. It hurt to hold my grandchildren after a few minutes—why, when I so enjoyed them tucked into my arms? It hurt to lie in bed or relax on the couch. It was the cross signaling of the sensory path with the pain path in the spinal column that often occurs in neurological disease. As my pathways strengthened the pain went away!

In January 2008, Dr. Brooks stated to our family, "You saw what your mother had been through and might be your future, you asked all the right questions, and then you went on to find the answers. Do not stop what you are doing! And share your knowledge."

It is now 2011 and I have made another leap to wellness. In 2010 my selegiline medication was changed to the patch form, EM-SAM. The medication is now constant in my system, no more "down" time. With this came an ability to move more freely with a higher energy. My husband enrolled us both in a gym. I started very slowly—at the simplest, but I saw the results very quickly. It wasn't that I had been lazy. I just needed the right medication and instruction. I was able to relearn how to move my arms and legs correctly with the machines to guide me. The strength training has helped to realign my posture. Exercising has led to reduced stress and better thinking and problem solving. I can feel the connection between my brain and my muscles. I have improved my balance and am less afraid of falling. Another huge improvement!

My support system of family, including my husband Wade, Cassie and Ken, Al and Erika, with grandchildren Max, Rosie and Shen, and friends is strong. It has expanded to all the wonderful people I meet through *forMemory*. As the primary founder and the President of *forMemory*, Inc., I have had the honor of speaking on behalf of those of us with early cognitive changes at numerous local, national and international conferences. I know that my words to scientists and to the public are an important part of making a difference for my children, grandchildren, and many people like myself. In sharing we are empowered by knowledge, taking away the destructive fear and replacing it with our identity, dignity and future. We are each unique. But we learn from each other. We seek wisdom for our own survival. We seek ways of prevention for others.

It has taken many years to regain much of my quality of life, with plenty of backward steps. I am surprised at each step forward. I am not cured, but healing, relearning how to love and to live.

I am a Survivor . . .

I am the contact for *forMemory* and its Data Base, Speaker's Bureau, "Time for Us" youth camp, and researchers.

Reach me at 821 West Browning St., Appleton, WI 54914, telephone (920) 734-9638 or email cbvanryzin@aol.com

Hope for the Future

Mary Kay Baum

In 2000 at the age of 52 I was ordained as a Lutheran pastor. I had excelled in theology, my second advanced degree. I had long ago completed law school. I had already been a community organizer, lawyer, law educator, manager of a neighborhood center network, school board member, county board member, and had run for mayor of Madison, Wisconsin. I was leading Madison-area Urban Ministry, a long-standing social justice non-profit, into new initiatives of working with persons who were formerly incarcerated. Since I was older than my sister, Chris Van Ryzin, who was battling serious confusion, and since I had no memory problems, I thought I had ducked the Alzheimer's/vascular dementia that frequented my mother's side of the family. But in my early 50's I was suddenly falling a lot. The UW Falls Clinic gave me advice on avoiding bifocals while walking, using a walking stick, and slowing down. I told them my mother and an aunt had died in their mid-seventies of Alzheimer's. We talked about how falling might link to early compromises in my brain. I have a health history of fainting, low blood pressure, low blood sugar and low iron count.

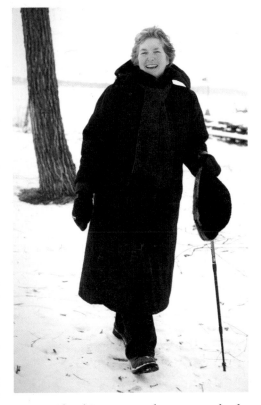

Our cross-generational research neurologist, Dr. Benjamin Brooks, was monitoring me because I had been having tremors, vertigo, and a second visual aura for no apparent reason. An EEG showed seizure activity near my language lobe and an MRI showed lesions in the same area. Dr. Brooks tracked and treated my subtle physical changes in circulation, reflexes, gait, grip, breath and strength well before my cognitive changes were measurable. He ordered a sleep study due to new problems with sleep disturbance. My sister, Chris, showed me hope for a future without the more serious symptoms that Alzheimer's usually brings.

The Wisconsin Alzheimer's Institute recently reported that small blood vessel disease with white matter changes can lead to the most common, costly, under-recognized, yet possibly most preventable cause of cognitive impairment. Not being able to find words is common early on. Now that this more general form of mild cognitive change is being recognized, doctors are asked to pay attention if a patient admits months after a stroke or a fall that she just isn't her old self anymore. Treating early symptoms is important for small blood vessel disease, Alzheimer's, or a combination of the two as in our family.

After a couple years of neuropsychological exams (called "normal" when compared to educated people of my age), I had one at age 57 that showed my verbal short-term memory was decreasing. It fit my own instinct. I was fatigued and became irritated with clients. When I could no longer get the words out to easily give instructions, I stayed late to do the work myself. I frequently lost my train of thought. The stress and long hours I was devoting to my work at the Madison-area Urban Ministry contributed to speeding my symptoms. I retired early from the work I loved in January 2006.

I believe I would not be speaking or living independently today if my seizure activity had not been dealt with while it was still sub-clinical, that is not observable. Now epilepsy specialists say my EEG's are "dreadful." That is, I would now be having frequent grand mal seizures if I were not on anti-seizure medication. My mother had frequent grand mal seizures and every time she had one she lost cognitively in a big way. It seems I have never had a seizure, not even a mini seizure. I was protected by early medication that was regularily adjusted upward to meet my needs. Dr. Brooks had gone the extra mile to order an EEG the first time I had an unex-plainable visual aura with no headache. This aura could have been from any number of reasons. I had almost ignored the one hour aura as people get them all the time, just I had never had one. And my HMO had al-ready ruled out any retina problem. This is my lesson for the public. Have any new, possibly neurological symptom checked out, especially if it could be a sign of early seizure activity. And my strong request to scientists and to practitioners is to order the relatively inexpensive and non-invasive EEG every couple years for anyone being tested for cog-nitive or neurological changes. Only a few practitioners are aware of links between Alzheimer's disease and seizures. The most recent study was in the UK and showed the incidence rate of seizures was 6.4 times higher for Alzheimer's patients than the public, and the younger the patient the more likely they were having seizures. This study was presented at the International Confer-ence on Alzheimer's Disease (ICAD) in Hawaii in 2010. Preventing damage to the brain from seizures is an important con-sideration in reducing the risk of full-fledged dementia.

I have moved to a rural housing coopera-tive amongst the oaks and prairies of south-west Wisconsin and am about 63 years old. I am the secretary and fund development chair for *forMemory*, Inc. I was recently hon-ored as a Wisconsin "Social Innovation Prize Fellow," living proof that the second half of life can be the most creative. I'll never again be the highly energetic public office holder and quick debater I used to be. I have fatigue after two hours of doing anything, especially social. I must pace myself and avoid crowds. I am easily distracted and therefore late for appointments. I get headaches from MSG, artificial sweeteners, and fabric softener. I have found taking melatonin and being in my own cool room helps me sleep soundly. I use organic fruits and vegetables and grass-fed animal products. I supplement with fish oil, herbs, and apoaequorin. I stay on my anti-seizure and ischemic meds. I have suc-cess with a selegiline patch both for depres-sion and for Parkinsonian-type symptoms of tremor and super flexed toes. I benefit from craniosacral therapy.

I now hike our hilly woods again. The more I hike the easier it seems to find words. My new adventure with photography is also a meditative break from over-stimula-tion. Working with others toward document-ing and restoring nature gives me immedi-ate goals.

I see now that my whole life has prepared me well for my calling to promote aware-ness and hope for memory. Even more pow-erful than memory is the power to hope for a healthy world and to connect with others to build that future of wellbeing for all ecosystems and communities.

When my framed nature photographs are not on exhibit elsewhere they hang in local assisted living communities. You can also see some of them at www.hopeofalzheimers .com. They are frequently premiums for do-nations to *forMemory*, Inc. I am happy to be contacted by mail at 3819 Evans Quarry Rd., Dodgeville, WI 53533, through email at mary kbaum@gmail.com or by phone at (608) 935-5834. Together we build hope for the future.

The Little Sister Who Cares

Rosann Baum Milius

I was raised on a dairy farm in the town of Grand Chute, which is located on the outskirts of Appleton, Wisconsin. I am number eight of nine Baum children, the "little sister."

I was eleven in 1970 when my mother started her earliest neurological symptoms at the age of 51. As my mother needed more care in 1976, I became one of her care providers, as she progressed through Alzheimer's disease and vascular dementia until her death in 1995 at age 75.

For many years I was looking at the disease from the outside. I became care partners with my two older sisters, Chris and Mary Kay, as their neurological symptoms evolved. Now, at the age of 51 I am personally dealing with my own cognitive changes.

For 20 years I held a senior level operations manager position for a multinational corporation. I was involved with hiring, training and developing account managers, supervisors and managers on sales and support teams for up to 120 people. After 20 years I became more stressed with the high demands of a large staff reporting to me and meeting our client expectations.

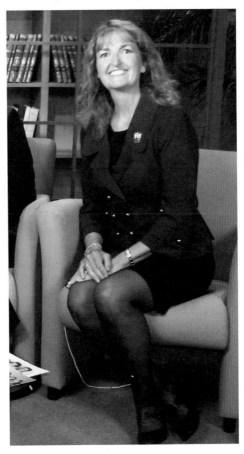

When a reorganization opportunity arrived I took a senior level client services role. In this position I focused on client relationships and financial data with most tasks completed in the quiet of my office. Even though I had no one reporting directly to me, it was still a very demanding role. Through the next three years my cognitive challenges increased and I had to work longer hours to complete work that would have been accomplished quite quickly in prior years. I taught myself to compensate for my cognitive changes but in 2009 I had to retire early after 23 years of service at the age of 50 with MCI–Mild Cognitive Impairment.

From 2000 to 2009 I volunteered on the board of directors for a local non-profit glass art museum. I served as Vice President for two years and then served as President of the Board for two years. I also chaired numerous committees. I left my board position in 2009, but I do continue to volunteer for the museum as my energy allows.

Since my early retirement I have focused on my health. I emphasize exercise (including running and yoga), good nutrition (including herbs and supplements), stress reduction, rest, mental stimulation, spirituality, and a positive attitude, all in my quest to keep my health from decreasing.

I advocate proactively to build a health and wellness team. Our bodies and brains are very complicated so I see numerous neurologists, doctors, researchers, and integra-

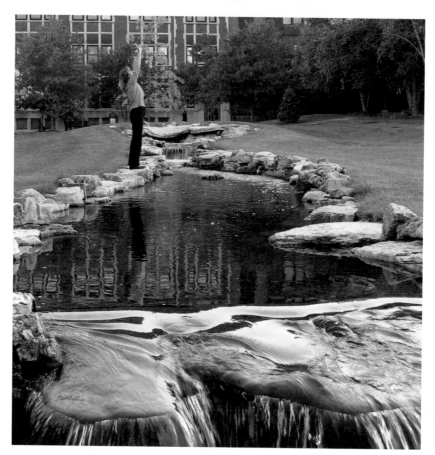

tive and holistic practitioners. Each has a different focus or specialty. I know that I am the foundation of my own health. I document changes that I experience with those on my health and wellness team. I have a health and wellness binder in which I place the purpose, contact information and photos of each practitioner and their administrative assistants. In this way I can find what I need quickly without the stress of looking through scattered papers. Also, if my husband or a care partner needs the information it will be easily available.

The knowledge gained from others on similar paths is invaluable. Increasing knowledge eliminates fear. I am an active member of *forMemory* and currently serve as Treasurer. Every member holds pieces to the puzzle so sharing symptoms, including what is and isn't working, is vital. There is so much information out there to read, research, and try.

I am deeply grateful for years of research and investigation that my sister Chris Baum Van Ryzin has documented. Being the "little sister" of both Chris and Mary Kay and gleaning from both of their experiences has helped me immensely on my own journey.

If I were to change one thing about how society responds to cognitive changes, I would make sure that each of us would have a skilled advocate/coordinator ready to guide us. My sisters were able to do some of this for me. But I think of all those not getting the early interventions they need because they have no idea of what to do or where to go. This resource could reduce frustration and costs.

For myself, I continue to provide care and support to family and friends. I consider this my true vocation. My mother taught us the art of TLC; tender, loving care. I do not have a nursing degree like my mother, but by being a care partner I feel I am following in my mother's footsteps.

I am married and live with my supportive and caring husband Doug in Oshkosh, Wisconsin. I am happy to be contacted by email at rosann.milius@gmail.com.

Like Something Out of Science Fiction

Chuck Jackson

I was diagnosed with Alzheimer's at age 50 in 2004. But I had strange occurrences long before that. I started documenting these happenings in my writings. There is great science fiction material in Alzheimer's!

I started falling when I first got out of bed. I was falling for no reason at all for at least two years before my diagnosis of Alzheimer's. It seemed that my brain forgot to tell my leg muscles that I was walking. Now some scientists are finally telling us that walking is a cognitive act that requires brain work. But most doctors still don't know that falling could have something to do with Alzheimer's, especially with someone who has a family history of early-onset Alzheimer's.

The same kind of thing was the disappearing tools. A tool would disappear right in front of me. I thought I was crazy. My brain just seemed to lose the tool's photographic image. My eye doctor could not diagnose me. He told me to see a mental health person.

Other early-onset people have admitted to me in hushed tones that they, too, experienced the "disappearing tools" thing. My earliest memory of my mother's Alzheimer's was her search for her glasses that were in plain sight for us. But she could not see them until I put them in her hand.

I was 13 years old when I was told of the Alzheimer's on my mother's side. I became my mother's caretaker when she was diagnosed in her early 40's. So I had already asked my family doctor about the earliest symptoms of the disease so I could watch for them. I was told, "We just don't know." It was only after I had started the meds and was talking with specialists about the disease that I found out that visual and motor problems are rather common in early Alzheimer's.

I learned in 2000 that I have a gene that would give me a 98 percent chance of getting Alzheimer's. Then, after 14 years of excellent reviews in my work as a nonprofit Employment Specialist, I received a bad job evaluation listing memory problems, poor organization, difficulty with speech, and be-

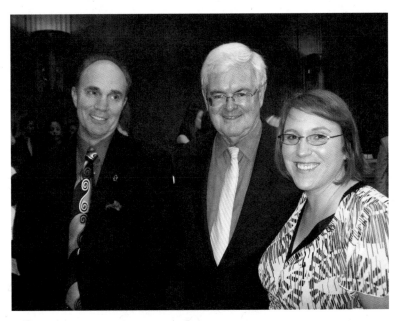

Chuck Jackson gave testimony to the Senate Special Committee on Aging in Washington, D.C. on May 14, 2008. Here he is pictured on the left with Newt Gingrich in the middle and Chuck's daughter Rachel Jackson on the right.

havioral problems. I once came to work wearing one black and one brown shoe. Asked to go home and change, I came back to the office wearing the other black shoe and brown shoe. This really annoyed my supervisor. I told my doctor about my job review, forgetting words, problems with muscle control, spasms of arms and legs, and the falling. My doctor said Alzheimer's had probably affected my brain and advised that I apply for disability benefits. I did so. I was fifty years old.I ask you, how can we report subtle changes if we don't know what to watch for? Scientists tell us now that by the time cognitive damage is measurable, a lot of damage has already been done. How can we get early treatment before serious cognitive damage if eye doctors, family doctors and psychologists don't ask about or even recognize early symptoms?

Most people think that to have Alzheimer's, you have to be brainless. Actually Alzheimer's is very subtle and sneaks up slowly. Even if you are like me, and have experience with other family members, you can still be surprised by what symptoms may appear.

I insist that more research focus on early symptoms. The findings should be published for all medical professionals and for the general public. Finally we need treatment . . . when we first experience what seem like science fiction events!

I currently live independently in Albany, Oregon with the help of my daughter and former wife. Seventeen of my relatives have died from Alzheimer's including my mother at age 50. My older brother and three cousins currently have Alzheimer's. I lead a monthly Early Stage Support Group, participate in research studies, and enjoy photography. See Resources on page 62 for a description of the highly reviewed book *The Thousand Mile Stare* that was written by my cousin in 2010 about our extended family and how we are living well with Alzheimer's.

You can hear more about my journey through the Story Corps radio project. Go to www.storycorps.net/listen/stories/charles-jackson.

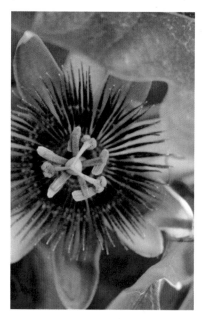

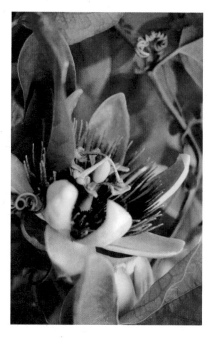

PHOTOS OF PASSIONFLOWER
BY CHARLES JACKSON
Notecards available. Contact Chuck at
balko71@yahoo.com

The Gift

Jim Cook

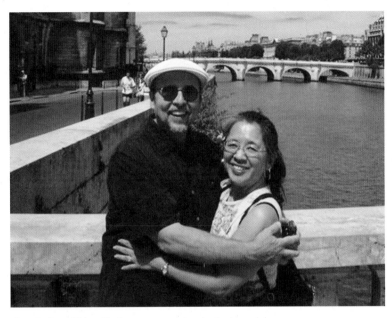

Jim Cook and his wife Gwen on vacation in Paris

I have a most unusual gift, the gift of "early knowing."

Just before my 56th birthday, an unexpected diagnosis dashed my vision of sparkling retirement filled with family and friends and travel, and crushed the time I assumed would be mine to express my many memories of an unusual life.

My diagnosis, early stage Alzheimer's disease, brought no immediate revulsion, just curiosity. Until that moment I had very little personal family experience with the "senility" of my elders. As one of the oldest of scores of grandchildren, I had many wonderful memories of my Great Plains grandparents and great-grandparents who had lived their long lives with seemingly intact mental abilities and remarkably good health. I assumed that same gift would follow for me and mine.

In the weeks following my Alzheimer's diagnosis, I sought information my wife Gwen and I would need to deal with this new disease. In what seemed a bitter irony, we had just completed a very difficult six-year period of direct caregiving for my mother, my grandmother and then my father, while also participating in long-distance caregiving for Gwen's brother and father. Now we faced another difficult caregiving experience. Uppermost was my concern for Gwen's health and well-being in the months and years ahead and this focus helped to defray my own sense of impending loss. Yet, as I reconciled myself to that loss of a hoped-for future, living in the moment now became a dominating force and led to the first hint of "my gift."

The year preceding my Alzheimer's diagnosis, I had—with some considerable reluctance—resigned my high-level university position. My position was created for me after I received two Master's Degrees from that same university—one in Community Planning and one from the Law School, while also concluding a 24-year Air Force career which included positions in medicine, flight training, engineering and journalism. Now, with this diagnosis, and considerable reflection, I came to believe that my resignation from the university was likely due in no small part to the behavior-related symptoms of my as-yet-undiagnosed early stage Alzheimer's disease.

I needed to know more, and learn more, from the experiences of others. I joined an Early Stage discussion group sponsored by my local Alzheimer's Association chapter, joined the chapter's Board of Directors and was invited to attend the Alzheimer's Association's National Forum in Washington D.C., where I spoke of my recent experiences after diagnosis with a presentation of "There's a Thief in my House."

My "gift of early knowing" was really the result of a series of events—an unexpected job loss, the unexpected illness of a sibling, my request for a "retirement physical" now that I was unemployed, and the expertise of my personal physician whose skill and inquisitiveness resulted in an MRI brain scan, indicating the likely presence of the disease. But for this sequence of events, my Alzheimer's disease would, even today, likely remain undiagnosed and untreated.

More importantly, without this early diagnosis, what I have learned about the disease and its progression would remain unknown to me, and the efforts to preserve my health and my future would not have been taken.

My gift is knowing, and from that knowing—action. I know I have a genetic predisposition for late onset of the disease with the double expression of APOE Allele 4, and that other co-morbidities including adult onset (type II) diabetes, obesity, metabolic syndrome, and chronic brain hypoxia from severe sleep apnea may be contributors to the existence and progression of my dementia. I work diligently to share this information and that some lifestyle choices may also be precursors to an early onset of dementia.

While attending that Washington D.C. Forum, Gwen and I met many others like us whose families also had an Early Stage diagnosis and experience, including the "for Memory" group. Chris Van Ryzin invited Gwen and me to attend *forMemory*'s inaugural national gathering the following month in Wisconsin. These two events were the first moments of my great awakening to the worldwide epidemic of Alzheimer's disease.

The gift of early knowing called me to get involved in creating awareness and learning what we could do to push back against Alzheimer's disease. I have recaptured some of the health of my youth through careful nutrition, aerobic activity, stress reduction, good sleep habits, the wise counsel of others, and lots of reading and research.

I served as an Advisor with the National Alzheimer's Association's Early Stage Advisory Group learning much from my colleagues and traveling widely to meet others in Town Hall forums, at professional conferences, and research centers. I remain active locally and nationally, adopting and sharing strategies to maintain good brain and body health—ideas and actions shared with others who are working with President Obama's administration to develop preventive strategies for the nation.

I have learned to attend to my health holistically, rather than to be pre-occupied with just Alzheimer's disease. Other health challenges can and will happen and it is those that deserve my focus today.

Trained as a planner, my hardest adjustment has been to live in the present. Preparing our home for the future is not as important as enjoying each day now. I wish for a quality future, but I focus on the present. The gift of knowing and attending to today is indeed a gift of life for the future.

———————

Jim and Gwen live in Lincoln, Nebraska near their family which includes seven grandchildren. Gwen manages an oral surgery practice and Jim seeks outlets in the arts, teaching, writing, and community involvement. They share a passion for their Hawaiian culture through nutritious luaus and an active hula troop. You can contact them through hulashack@gmail.com.

Transporting to New Hope

Charley Schneider

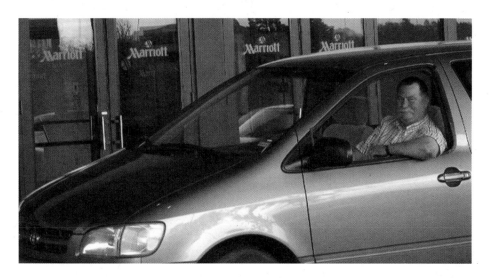

I was a firefighter, a police detective and a construction worker in St. Louis until I was diagnosed at age 52 with early-onset Alzheimer's disease. In my past work, I had transported nursing home residents with late-stage Alzheimer's disease to the ambulance or morgue. So when I was diagnosed with early-onset Alzheimer's disease I just assumed I would die very soon.

But then my wife, Barb, and I met other people with the same diagnosis and I learned new hope. Many who had been diagnosed eight or ten years ago were still going strong in their own way. Many were writing, communicating, advocating and traveling to meet with each other. I work with Dementia Advocacy and Support Network International (DASNI) and with *forMemory*.

After chatting with my own real peers and observing my own changes, it seems to me that attitude and will power actually slow down or expedite this disease's progress. I even wonder if Alzheimer's disease can be overcome indefinitely or at least until we die of unrelated causes. I think this may be possible. One thing I do know is that will power and hope sure don't hurt. And any unconditional love given to us serves as a powerful source for our own will power and hope.

I have two children and five grandchildren in the St. Louis area. I now realize that there are many reasons why it is beneficial to my loved ones and to others for me to live longer. I have written a book entitled *Don't Bury Me, It Aint Over Yet*. I want to help doctors, caregivers and persons with Alzheimer's disease to understand that this diagnosis is not necessarily a rapid death sentence. I feel that many people who are diagnosed with Alzheimer's give up in shame and fear. They allow the disease to rapidly overcome them. This kind of "false-hope-lessness" is deadly.

I am truly excited about the extended time I may have been given. Instead of planning for rapid decline and death, I have started again to plan future goals for my life.

I have dedicated the remainder of my life to promoting the early recognition, treatment and cure of dementia. I want to empower people with dementia and their families to live joyful and productive lives.

———————

You can contact me at
charley3rd@yahoo.com.

A Picture Worth 1,000 Words

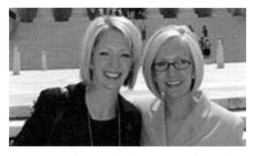

Melissa Washburn and Cambria Anderson

Cambria, Melissa and Katie's mother, Carol Anderson, died in 2008 at the age of 52."Through our mother we were given an understanding of the 'spirit of life'. We gained a deeper understanding of faith, hope and love. Ultimately her death taught us about the power of living. We have moved onto a protective, preventative approach to wellness aided by the continuing sharing of knowledge within our *forMemory* friends. Having knowledge is a gift. Having trust and faith in knowledge is powerful. We know that we can make a difference in our lives and those of our children. We already are!"

Here is our story as reported in 2006 at the Alzheimer's Association "Public Policy Forum Advocate Profile."

When their 46-year-old mother, Carol, was diagnosed with early-onset Alzheimer's disease, sisters Melissa Washburn and Cambria Anderson experienced a period of shock, sadness and mourning. How could someone so young, vibrant and in the prime of her life fall victim to this devastating disease, they wondered. Then, taking a page from their mother's own book, they decided such thinking wasn't going to do anyone any good, and they set out to learn as much as they could about the disease, its treatments and the possibility of a cure.

"Everything we do we do out of respect for our mom," said Cambria, now a 31-year-old mother of two from Idaho Falls, Idaho. "Our mom was a powerhouse. She sought answers when she needed them and she didn't take no for an answer."

The sisters' quest for answers led them to contact Alzheimer researchers, as participating in research was important to both mother and daughters.

"I think her background as a nurse made her willing to do it, and she saw it as a way to contribute to the scientific and medical community," recalled Melissa, a 29-year-old stay-at-home mom from Orem, Utah. The scarcity of early-onset trials, however, was frustrating for all. "Here was our mom saying, 'Study me,' but she didn't qualify for anything because she was too young."

And so the sisters emailed personal pleas to some of the world's most renowned Alzheimer researchers. Much to their surprise and delight, several responded, and as a result they were able to meet with researchers at the University of Washington and enroll their mom in a research study.

Their belief that hope lies in continued research led the sisters to register for the 2006 Alzheimer's Association Public Policy Forum—even though they had no prior advocacy experience. They did, however, have a powerful story to share.

The realization that their mom's story might be an effective advocacy tool came to them through the process of assembling a scrapbook of her life. They entered the book into a scrapbooking contest and ended up winning the $10,000 grand prize.

"What really took us to the next level of wanting to share our story with other people was how touched the judges were by the book and my mom's life. They had no idea Alzheimer's could strike someone so young," Melissa said. "They said, 'you have such a fantastic story to share, you've got to share it with other people.'"

And so last June, Melissa, Cambria, and their father, Mark, used the prize money to fly to Washington for the Forum. There, they realized for the first time that they weren't unique and there are many more people in the same boat. The bonds forged with those other early-onset families and caregivers remain strong today.

"We speak on the phone weekly and e-mail constantly. We created a network of support for each other in *forMemory*," Melissa said.

The sisters also remain in touch with many of the aides and legislators that they met during the Forum's lobbying session, something they credit to the lasting impact of their mom's early-onset story.

"A couple people said, 'I didn't even know this could happen.' And to me that just said, we have so much work to do if our own legislators don't know this can strike younger people," Melissa said. "Yes, it is exhausting, but there's so much to be motivated for. We know, for our mom, a cure was not possible, and even treatment was not an option at that point. But they are for us, and for our kids. How could we not do it?"

You may contact them at:
Melissa Washburn, 801-434-7758, sm_washburn@yahoo.com
Cambria Anderson, 208-357-3751, anderson44@ida.net

Living, Loving, Playing, Learning, and Contributing

Wantland J. (Jay) Smith

I was diagnosed with early Alzheimer's disease in late 2005, based on neuropsychological tests and a confirming FDG/PET scan. I had become disabled from work a year-and-a-half earlier due to fatigue—apparently caused by the extraordinary mental effort to overcompensate for my yet undiscovered memory problems. I now consider myself a "survivor," with ups and downs, but still living well while contributing to the well-being of those around me.

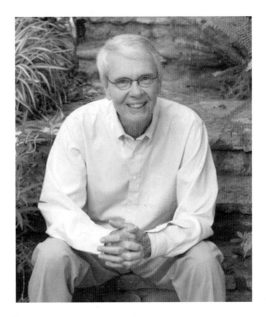

I take my Rx meds every day, all three of them—Exelon, Namenda, and Lipitor—and I believe they are helping me. The notion that the meds don't help people in the long run was based on studies done several years ago on older people who were more advanced in dementia, were conducted for just a few months, and weren't done on people taking the combination cocktail of drugs. I haven't seen any studies of younger people diagnosed with early Alzheimer's who took the drugs over a long period of time. A 9/2008 report of a study at Massachusetts General Hospital showed that people who took cholinesterase inhibitors in combination with Namenda (memantine) had a slower progression of the disease than those who took only one of the two drugs. So I'm taking my meds with some hope for the best. I believe they're keeping me going, with both good days and not so good ones.

But taking my medicine is not the only thing I am doing. Upon diagnosis over five years ago, I began reading about Alzheimer's and about general health. I was encouraged by what I had read by Deepak Choprah, Andrew Weil, Dharma Singh Khalsa, Dean Ornish, and especially the first Alzheimer's survival pioneer Morris Friedell, who was introduced to me by David Shenk's book, *The Forgetting*. I began to develop my own life-style approach. Eventually I put together a three-legged stool of lifestyle strategies.

The three parts of my strategy are 1) aerobic and mental exercise, 2) healthy diet and nutritional supplements, and 3) stress reduction or socialization.

1) Exercise is essential for physical health and for a healthy brain. Science has shown that aerobic exercise combined with learning something new is the foundation for our built-in process for building new neural pathways and growing brain mass. Regular physical exercise, coupled with consistently challenging mental activity, such as learning a new language or musical instrument, is key to a healthy body and brain. Music, plus daily sudoku and crossword puzzles are my main mental exercise activities.

2) Since going on disability nearly seven years ago, I've been adhering to a healthy Mediterranean diet that is mostly vegan. I'm taking several of the supplements listed in the recent NIA/NIH "2005–2006 Progress Report on Alzheimer's" as currently in clinical trials. I'm also taking several supplements recommended specifically for brain health, and for cardiovascular health.

3) My approach to socialization is guided by concepts of Dr. Ornish on "love and intimacy," Dr. Jon Kabat-Zinn on stress reduction, and Dr. Herbert Benson on relaxation. Many of my activities are music related, including mandolin playing, vocal lessons, and chorus. I stay connected to family and enjoy being with the grandchildren. I participate in early stage support groups, a social activity that gives me perspective about myself and provides me a chance to give back to others. I also believe that it is good for my health.

While conventional medicine does not have a lot to offer us in the way of treating Alzheimer's, other than the combination of approved medications, I believe there is so much we can do for ourselves. My patchwork quilt of strategies is made up from lots of separate pieces, each of which are thought to contribute to preventing the disease or to slowing its progression. Until we have more effective pharmaceutical treatments, this holistic approach is all we can do. A few practicing doctors are beginning to adopt the approach—giving me hope that it will eventually become mainstream. One of them, Dr. Kenneth Kosik at UC Santa Barbara, has opened a one-stop Alzheimer's treatment clinic that uses a range of conventional and alternate therapies.

In 2006, while developing a questionnaire on people's road to diagnosis and their earliest symptoms, I offered my prediction that one day we would be diagnosing people in the earliest stages of the disease, even in a stage of "no symptoms." I noted that this was the way to understand and find effective treatments and, ultimately, its cure. My prediction gained credence last summer at ICAD 2010, when leading researchers announced the NIA/Alzheimer's Association joint project for developing new diagnostic criteria for three stages of Alzheimer's disease. The earliest of the three stages is the preclinical stage that includes persons with either no symptoms or yet benign subjective symptoms.

Getting a diagnosis at an early stage can be liberating, as mine was. An early diagnosis allows people to plan their futures and make the lifestyle adjustments necessary to enjoy the years ahead. Those of us living with Alzheimer's disease don't see it as merely a clinical condition for which we are totally reliant on doctors for guidance. Rather, we strive to see it as being an opportunity for taking responsibility for ourselves, so we can enjoy living fully for as long as possible. I'm having a great time living, loving, playing, learning, and contributing.

I live with my wife, Marilyn, in Los Angeles. I can be reached for comments or speaking engagements through my email address at wantland.smith@sbcglobal.net.

Down a Different Path

Richard Taylor, Ph.D.

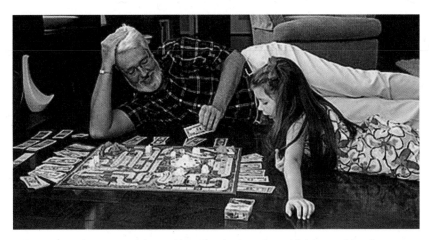

When not speaking around the world, Richard enjoys time with his granddaughter.

I am not only marching to a different drummer, but also marching down a different path. And I want to focus on today's path.

Too often you just want to remind me of my past, my old memories, and my yesterdays. That is not all that helpful. Instead I need to pay attention to today.

It's true that sometimes I do things "right" in the morning and "wrong" in the afternoon. I often recall details no one else does. I sometimes forget major points everyone else knows. My thinking varies day to day and hour to hour. Sometimes I improve several steps, and then find myself stepping backwards, or more likely, sideways.

If you unnecessarily take over my decisions, lay out my clothes, dress me, choose my groceries, order my food for me, then there is less and less for me to decide. Instead of making all my decisions for me, simply prompt me to make as many decisions as possible. Give me cues or a memory aid to encourage me to live fully in today.

More than pharmaceuticals, we need "socialceuticals." We need innovative and adaptive models of how to live with the symptoms, how to live with ourselves, how to live with others.

In the eyes of many I am seen as less than a complete someone. In my own eyes I am still a whole and complete someone. I am still grandpa, and dad, a friend, and a whole human being. I have always been a complete person and I still am. I am not becoming any less a person simply because I cannot remember exactly like you do, talk like you do, or think like you do.

It is true that I am fundamentally different from you. I am different in ways I can't express and you can't fully perceive or understand. Our brains are different. But I am still a complete human being. I am marching to a different drummer and down a different path than you. But I am still me and it is still today.

Richard Taylor, a retired psychologist, was diagnosed with probable Alzheimer's at age 58. Now 66, he lives with his spouse Linda in Cypress, Texas. His son and family live across the street. Richard authored the book, *Alzheimer's From the Inside Out* (Health Professions Press, 2007) to describe his progression through early stages of Alzheimer's. Richard's Newsletter is found at www.richardtaylorphd.com. His email to arrange speaking is richardtaylor @gmail.com.

On My Way to Better Health

Karen Waterhouse

I was diagnosed with early-onset Alzheimer's disease in August of 2005 and started on Aricept and Namenda. I left my stressful high-level government accounting job.

I am a socially active person with a supportive family. My husband John and I became involved with the Alzheimer's Association in St. Louis and attend monthly meetings to help us live with the disease.

In June 2006 the Alzheimer's Association asked us to go to Washington D.C. for the Alzheimer's Public Policy Forum. It helped turn my life around because I met other people there who also had early-onset Alzheimer's disease! We were able to talk directly with each other about how we were living with these challenges. We compared notes about our backgrounds and about what seemed to help us now.

While at the forum I met Chris Baum Van Ryzin who wrote a book about her experiences, entitled *Alzheimer's Averted*. Reading her story inspired me to explore nutrition and herbs to complement my prescribed medications. I researched herbs that tend to reduce inflammation. Using herbs as supplements and in bath water has made me feel much better. An Alzeimer's Association spirituality class enhances my life overall.

I read an article that said that Alzheimer's disease is very rare in India, and that it could be because they use turmeric in cooking. I spoke with my doctor about using it in my food, and he said it would be very good for me and could be helpful for memory. So I have added turmeric to something I eat every day.

I also eat healthy, using plenty of fresh fruits and vegetables daily, avoiding foods containing monosodium glutamate, and taking omega-3's and other vitamins daily. I try to avoid the toxins in the water, air, food and environment.

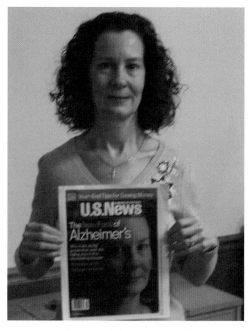

Karen Waterhouse and the Dec. 3, 2006 U.S. News & World Report which features Karen when she was 50 years old, one year after her diagnosis.

I stay very busy working my brain daily through crossword puzzles, find-a-word puzzles, Sudoku puzzles, and books. Often when I start reading a new book, I have to take notes to help me understand the plot. I watch the news to keep current with world events. I continue to enjoy various creative arts including needlework. My husband and I walk 45 minutes daily for exercise. My balance and stamina keep on improving.

I had my annual checkup in October of 2008 with my neurologist at Washington University Memory Diagnostic Center in St. Louis. He told me that I had actually improved from last year on my test scores. He was very pleased with this. He told me to definitely continue doing all the things I am currently doing.

I now have test results and a neurologist saying I'm improving my health! I hope others will pay attention to supplements, herbs, nutrition, exercise, mental stimulation and the environment as ways to better health.

Contact me at John63303@netscape.net.

My Alzheimer's Story

Darryl White

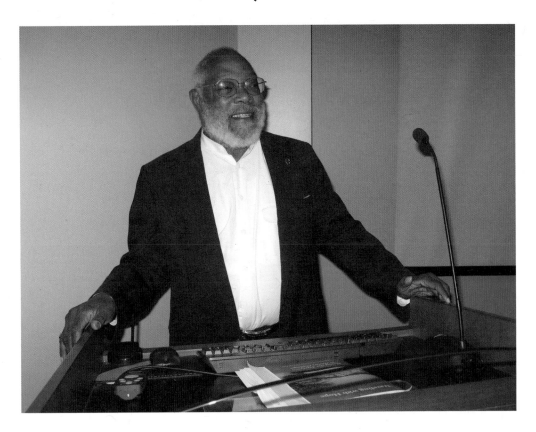

I was in my early to mid 50's when my mother was diagnosed with Alzheimer's. Then when I was 61, my wife and I were preparing to dine out in celebration of our 38th wedding anniversary when I received a phone call from California. My sister told me that my mother had just died due to her Alzheimer's.

I had been diagnosed with early stage Alzheimer's several years after I learned of my mother's Alzheimer's diagnosis. I was employed as a State of Wisconsin Probation and Parole Agent in downtown Madison when diagnosed. I was eventually forced to leave this work.

I really wanted to continue my job with accommodations as specified for some conditions under disability law. I discussed options like voice-generated documents, smaller caseload, and other accommodations to help me complete reports. My office had insufficient clerical workers for the number of agents assigned to the office and timeliness of written reports is a significant factor in how parole officers are evaluated. My employer did not offer me accommodations.

With my life experiences as an African American male, I know I could have continued to positively affect others, especially young African American men, who represented a high percentage of my case load. But, in a letter I received from my employer, I was told that due to my diagnosis with dementia I was no longer able to perform the duties of employment as an agent of the state of Wisconsin.

When I first joined Alzheimer's work it was primarily to help me deal with issues of my mother's diagnosis, with her living in California with family and me in Wisconsin. More recently, I joined the Alzheimer's & Dementia Alliance of Wisconsin (ADAW) to advocate for the issues of all who have a dementia diagnosis. We advocate with elected legislative, state, and federal officials. We advocate with State of Wisconsin employment officials to urge them to make accommodations for others in our situations, now and in the future. I continue to benefit from ADAW's Crossing Bridges support and Meeting of the Minds activities. In 2009 I received the "Courage in Advocacy" award from the Wisconsin State Alzheimer's conference.

National Press

In February 2008 I was interviewed by *USA Today* about a survey conducted for the Alzheimer's Association and the American Heart Association during Black History Month about combined risk factors. As an African American I am more at risk for diabetes and other cardiovascular problems. What I said in the article was that I had no idea that diabetes and other cardiovascular problems put me at more risk for Alzheimer's. I was like most African Americans in the survey in that I did not realize that high blood pressure and high cholesterol increase the risk for Alzheimer's, not just for heart attack and stroke. In this 2007 survey one-third of black Americans reported having a diagnosis of high blood pressure; about one in five said they had high blood cholesterol. More than half of the African-Americans had realized that such factors put them at higher risk of having a heart attack or a stroke, but just 8% realized such conditions also put them at a greater risk of dementia.

State Press

In May of 2008, through coordination with the Alzheimer's Association, my wife, Bridget, and I traveled to Washington, D.C. We helped educate lawmakers about many memory loss issues. We told them about our needs for more research and better treatment options. While in Washington in conjunction with Senator Kohl's congressional hearing on aging we were interviewed by the *Milwaukee Journal Sentinel*. In response to the reporter's questions I explained how I sometimes forget things. I said I have trouble concentrating on a task at hand, like sometimes paying our bills on time.

On occasion in talking, I have to say, "Where was I going with that?" when I lose my chain of thought.

I recommended the movie "The Notebook," about a man who visits his ailing wife in a nursing home and reads their love story to her even though she often cannot remember him as her husband and is sometimes upset with his caring demeanor.

When I lost my way in telling my story for the Milwaukee paper, my wife Bridget intervened, speaking up and helping me get back on track. However, she went on to say that she worries I would one day forget who she is. I told her, in front the reporter, "I'll always know who you are."

Local Press

I was interviewed by *The Madison Times* after speaking to a group primarily of members of the African American community at their South Side Center. I told my story about how both my mother and aunt were diagnosed with Alzheimer's. I explained that high blood pressure and high cholesterol increase the risk for Alzheimer's, not just for heart attack and stroke. Diabetes that many of us persons of color have is also a risk factor for Alzheimer's. I said I wish I had gotten the message earlier. If I had known earlier, I might have made more of a point of continuing to exercise and watching my diet to prevent my midlife weight gain, diabetes, and high blood pressure. I may still have developed the disease. But I wondered aloud whether with those precautions I just might have delayed it long enough to continue working years longer in my chosen profession. I did not take these precautions soon enough. If it is too late for me, it may not be for those in the audience.

Current Initiatives

We now know that African Americans are two times more likely to develop Alzheimer's disease than Caucasians. This is partly due to the fact that we are more likely to develop diabetes, high blood pressure and high cholesterol, all of which are known risk factors for dementia. We have also been disproportionately affected for generations by toxic environments, under-attention, and lack of access to preventive healthcare.

African Americans often cope in silence without access to prevention strategies, interventions, resources or treatment. ADAW is the first Alzheimer's organization in the nation to have a diversity coordinator (Charlestine Daniel) linking the African American community to researchers at an NIH-funded Alzheimer's Disease Research Center.

There are also historical reasons why the African American community is skeptical of researchers. Trust will need to be built back slowly in order to raise the comfort level enough for people to consider participating in studies.

The ADAW is hosting a Carter Fuller Day memory screening at our local Urban League. Dr. Solomon Carter Fuller was the first black psychiatrist in the United States and played a key role in the development of psychiatry in the 1900s. Dr. Carter Fuller worked closely with Dr. Alois Alzheimer, the namesake of Alzheimer's disease.

My wife and I continue to advocate each spring in Washington, DC with our Wisconsin delegation in Congress.

Together may we empower diverse and forgotten populations to experience hope for the future.

I can be contacted at
darryl_white@uwalumni.com.

In This Moment . . . In This Day . . .
A New Chance to Live

Dee Cauble

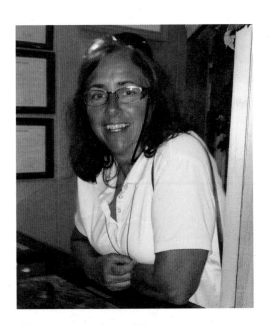

It was in 2009, when my two sisters and I attended a presentation at Bellin Health in Green Bay, Wisconsin. The topic was on attaining a higher quality of life with early onset cognitive challenges and it was here that we were introduced to the *forMemory* organization. After the presentation my sisters and I stayed to talk with Chris Van Ryzin, the speaker. She answered my questions and listened to my fears. She invited me to attend her community outreach group the next day on my way back home to Minnesota where each month they research another aspect of wellness.

I am married to Bruce and have three children; two are in college and one teenager. We live in Edina, Minnesota outside of Minneapolis. I earned a Bachelor of Science degree with a double major in Rehabilitation and Human Relations with a concentration on Psychology from the University of Wisconsin–Stout. Through my work I developed many skills including leadership, project management of multi-faceted and time driven projects, production coordinator, sales team leader, marketing and promotions, and coordinating events.

I was a stay at home mother for our three children. As they grew, I started a new career in real estate. I earned my real estate broker license and ran my own business from 2004 to 2007.

When I reached my late 40's I began to experience cognitive challenges, which caused me to leave my real estate business. Everything took so much longer to do. I felt like I was spinning my wheels. I could not complete the tasks I started. This is what led me to the talk at Bellin Health that night.

Chris and I talked of the Time for Us camp for my son that summer, but it took one more year to "make it happen." Even then it was taking some creative thinking to get our son Connor to Elkhorn in lower Wisconsin from the Minneapolis area. One by one the available options we tried were crossed off the list. It was decided that I should attend with our son as a volunteer helper. The two of us could drive down together, each supporting the other, as a team. A new concept for a mother/son, but now needed.

As the camp days went by, it was clearly seen that both of us were benefiting from the Time for Us camp. We grew in an awareness and hope, developing a new determination to take charge, finding that there are positive steps to be taken. And that this does not have to be a quick trip—but a long, fulfilling path. The days provided a good balance between interaction and respite with companionship for us both, as the *forMemory* volunteer directors also share memory/cognitive challenges. Having a new volunteer "job" after so much loss, gave me my dignity back. We both tried new ideas. Being able to voice for the first time his concerns for me and being understood, brought relief to Connor.

In sharing, it was realized that my path may have started differently. We do not have a strong history of cognitive changes in my family. I did, however, suffer from numerous injuries to my head as a youth and an adult. Because of that, I sought out and found a neurologist who specializes in brain injuries whom I have added to my health care team. I am also working on integrative aspects to wellness. The times that I can find my words and my memory is the best, is when I am walking with my girlfriends.

What I feel is most important is to have others to talk to who are experiencing like symptoms. There is a support group for my husband, as a care partner, but not yet for any of the young onset in our home area. I hope one day to be able to make that change.

I would love to hear from others in my community. deecauble@pobox.com

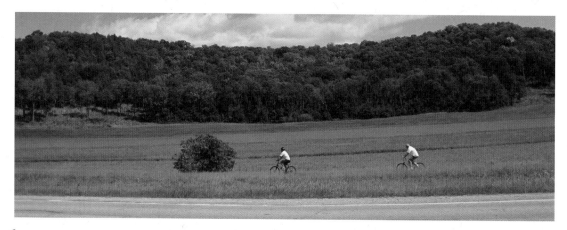

III. *forMemory and Its Projects*

"It's good just to feel like we're moving forward.
And something else, just simply the camaraderie in our peer group.
We all agree that the very first time we found others like ourselves
to talk to it was amazing. It was like finding a jewel."

—*Charley Schneider, Board of Directors of forMemory, Inc.*

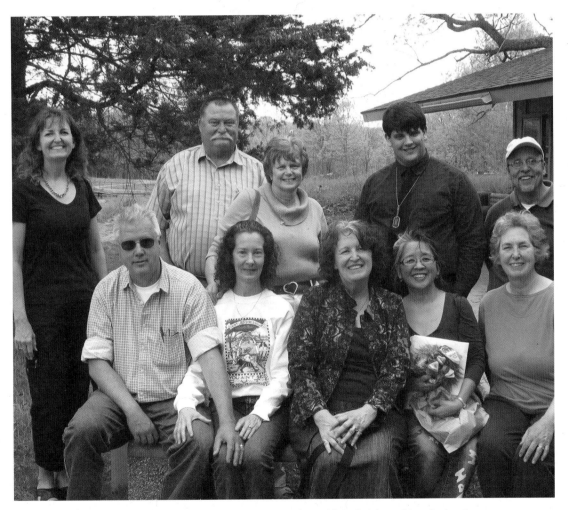

Our Board of Directors and many care partners presented, provided a booth, and met during the 2010 Wisconsin State Alzheimer's and Related Disorders Conference. Jim Cook delivered the closing keynote at the conference. Another highlight was the visit to the International Crane Foundation in nearby Baraboo. Shown there are (back row) Rosann Milius, Charley and Barbara Schneider and their grandson Christopher, and Jim Cook; (front row) John and Karen Waterhouse, Chris Van Ryzin, Gwen Cook, and Mary Kay Baum.

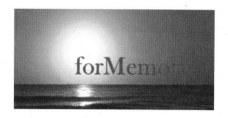

Building Hope
in Early Onset Alzheimer's
and Related Diseases

Mission

The mission of *forMemory* is to bring together those of us affected directly or indirectly by early onset Alzheimer's and related diseases to increase our emotional, spiritual, and physical well-being through actively and aggressively seeking ways of healing and preventing early onset neurodegenerative disorders.

Goals

Replace Aloneness with Hope

We are not alone: "Call me. I will listen. I understand."
Empower each other through our emotional support.

Replace Fear with Knowledge

We each are holding some of the pieces to the whole picture.
Because of early diagnosis, we are still able to communicate.
Share the ideas that are working to reduce symptoms: "I feel better when . . ."

Replace Disease with Life

Aggressively seek new information by looking outside the box.
Actively seek, learn, compare and research.
Partner with doctors and researchers.
Make genetic testing available for those who desire it.
Consider the whole person—mind, body, and spirit.

Replace Silence with a United Voice

Speak out in a united voice.
We who have early-onset cognitive changes have the strongest voices . . . for those who no longer can speak.
By sharing our experiences we improve our quality of life and that of our families.

Activities

We are meeting regularly to share and increase our knowledge. We document and have available for persons or researchers our earliest symptoms, what makes us better, and what makes us worse. We discuss environmental, nutritional and stress-related influences. Through maintaining an informational web site for communication we share the information on early-onset with others affected by dementia diseases so they may also benefit. We provide training and materials nationwide for congregations and civic groups on ways to support and empower persons or families with early-onset cognitive changes. We helped to establish services for midwest youth including a five day Time for Us camp for teens whose lives are touched by dementia. By speaking out as a united voice, we build hope in early-onset Alzheimer's and related diseases.

Special thoughts from very hopeful families.

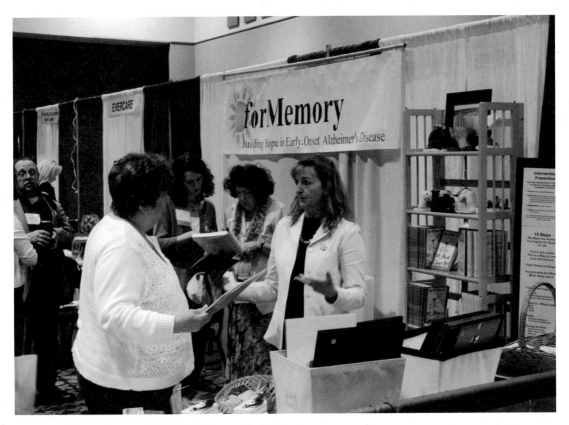

Our volunteers set up and staff a forMemory display booth at many conferences.

We are persons affected directly or indirectly by Alzheimer's or related challenges whose symptoms started before the age of 65 years (early onset). We advocate for a partnership in accessible health care and research systems, community connectedness, and a planet free of toxins. We have a passion to improve the quality of life for ourselves, our children, and future generations worldwide. Activities include research collaboration on a database, a camp for youth impacted, peer support, education and outreach.

Our first national meeting was held in conjunction with Wisconsin State Alzheimer's Conference in 2007. We gained our not-for-profit tax-exempt certification on April 12, 2010. Our officers are: Chris Baum Van Ryzin (Wisconsin), President; James M. Cook (Nebraska), Vice President; Mary Kay Baum, (Wisconsin) Secretary; Rosann Milius (Wisconsin), Treasurer; and Cambria Anderson (Idaho), Committee Leader. Additional Board Members are Charley Schneider (Missouri) and Karen Waterhouse (Missouri).

Volunteers include: Mark Anderson, Alice Bartel, Bonnie Benson, Rich Bozanich, Bill Bridgwater, Dee and Bruce Cauble, Casandra and Ken Cobb, Gwendolyn Cook, Rosemary Counard, Charlie Daniel, Mike Donohue, Sue and Gene Eckes, Stephanie Flenz, Mary Friedel-Hunt, Tom Fritsch, Caroline Hoffman, Chuck Jackson, Mona Johnson, Jaye Lander, Mary Ann McKenna, Doug Milius, Carole Mulliken, Cynthia Mochel, Jane Rundell, Barb Schneider, Josh Shapiro, Dan and Gina Smith, Wantland "Jay" and Marilyn Smith, Mike Soletski, Catherine Stephens, George and Jake Swamp, Richard Taylor, Wade Van Ryzin, Melissa Washburn, John Waterhouse, Darryl and Bridget White and many others who share pathways of hope.

forMemory Database:
A Hopeful Collaboration

It started in conversation. By talking with each other, *forMemory* realized that those of us with memory challenges also had physical problems. The more we talked, the more we realized that many of us had *similar* physical symptoms. Then looking back together, we realized that the physical changes preceded noticeable memory loss.

We felt we might be on to something. Shouldn't we document this anecdotal discovery and see how real it was? Even in our families with early-onset histories, no doctors had told us to watch for subtle physical changes. Our physicians had not given us examples of changes that might have the potential of being neurological symptoms.

Early changes for most of us included two or three of the following: fatigue, tremor, weakness, vertigo, leg pain, falling, irritability, loss of coordination and/or disturbed sleep. Many of us had changes in our spatial awareness, gait and/or eyesight. A few of us had for the first times in our lives experienced heart palpitations, bright light auras or other possible signs of mild seizure activity.

Most of us have a relative or two with dementia. Our relatives may have had neurological changes in their early stages. But nobody seemed to connect it to their dementia. Even today many physicians would not know to watch for possible "markers" across generational lines in affected families.

So *forMemory* initiated a project for gathering data from persons in all stages of memory loss. Mona Johnson, known for her The Tangled Neuron website, drafted our first database instrument. We encouraged using calendars to pay attention to ongoing patterns. We hoped for data to include demographics, early changes, test results, environmental histories, other illnesses, and reactions to chemicals such as pesticides and food additives. We also wanted anecdotal reports on what was enhancing quality of life such as physical activity, medications, supplements, anti-inflammatory herbs, physical therapy, creative arts, massage, oils, etc.

We wanted a well-designed database protocol that would incorporate confidentiality. Our test database was developed with the assistance of research neurologist Dr. Benjamin Rix Brooks and researcher Craig S. Atwood, Ph.D.

Dr Atwood says, "I credit *forMemory* for their foresight to begin to gather the epidemiological data that is needed to direct

We were honored to present a poster at the International Conference on Alzheimer's Disease in July 2008 on our "Hopeful Collaboration: Scientists & Persons with Memory Loss Work Together to Provide Hope through a Research-Oriented Database."

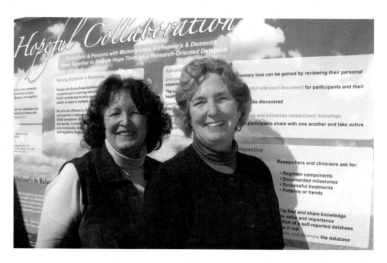

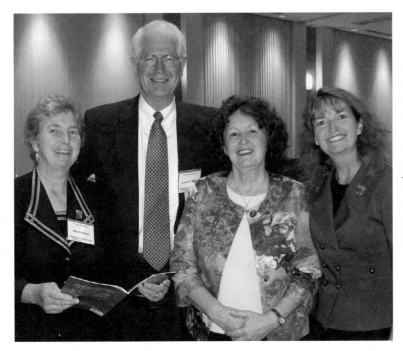

The Baum sisters updated Dr. John C. Morris, MD, director of Washington University's Knight Alzheimer's Disease Research Center, on the forMemory database during WU's 2009 Leonard Berg Symposium on presymptomatic detection of dominantly inherited Alzheimer's disease.

future research at the biological and clinical levels. Scientific assessment of what is helping them will lead to exciting new avenues for therapeutics."

We have already noticed that many of us are exploring paths of complementary medicine. Examples are as diverse as coconut oil, vitamin E, B vitamins, and Gotu Kola.

Some use bio-identical hormone replacement therapy. Others of us have been tested and receive prescriptions to prevent silent seizure activity. Some receive prescriptions for Eldepryl, also known as Selegiline. While approved by the FDA here for our Parkinsonian symptoms and depression, in Europe Eldepryl is also prescribed more generally for early Alzheimer's disease.

The process of completing the questionnaire prompts us to think about our own experiences in new ways and leads us to discuss additional therapies with our physicians. A database does not take the place of our physicians and we always talk over any symptoms and therapies with them.

Similar self-reporting databases have been established for diseases like Parkinson's and endometriosis to help in the development of new therapies.

Our database was initiated by those of us with early memory challenges so the patterns we are experiencing will likely be detected. We won't overlook clues that could benefit our families and future generations. We commit to updating our database information annually. We commit ourselves to encouraging others to participate.

We always hoped to find an accredited research institution to take up the protocols and test database that we had initiated. We are happy that Craig S. Atwood, Ph.D. through the Laboratory of Endocrinology, Aging and Disease (LEAD) has agreed to do so. LEAD plans to refine the database questionnaire, meet institutional and scientific standards, collect the data on a website of their own, and maintain participant confidentiality. Over time LEAD will conduct analyses of data to provide scientifically valuable information.

We realize that by providing LEAD with our first-hand observations contributes to the understanding, prevention, and early treatment of Alzheimer's and related dementias. Visit LEAD's preliminary website at *www.formemorydatabase.org* to find out more about this truly hopeful collaboration.

TIME FOR US

A Midwest summer camp for young teens who are connected to someone with a memory, cognitive, or neurological challenge

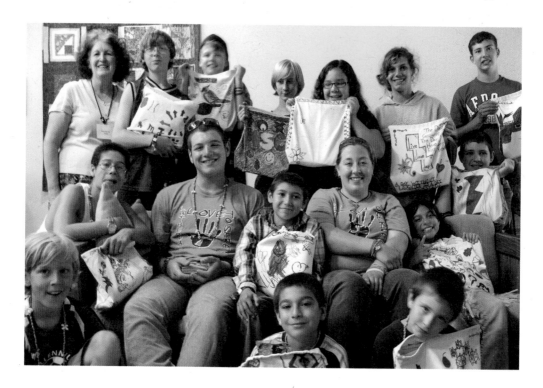

What is it about?

TIME FOR US is a great camping opportunity for teens from 11 to 17 years of age who have a loved one with a neurological challenge including Alzheimer's disease or a similar memory/cognitive challenge. Most of each day is spent on fun camp activities—ropes challenge, tower climbing, canoeing, water sports, field sports, etc. In addition a portion of each day focuses on a healthy brain including an understanding of cognitive and memory challenges through a unique Keeper of Memories program. Campers who attended the camp say it was "Great!"—are coming back and bringing siblings!

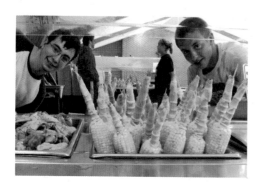

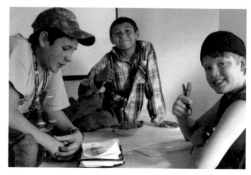

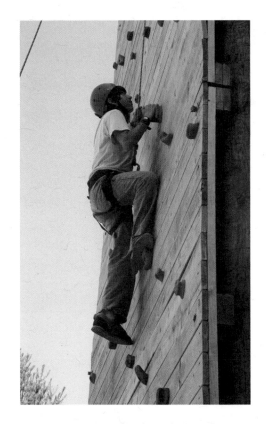

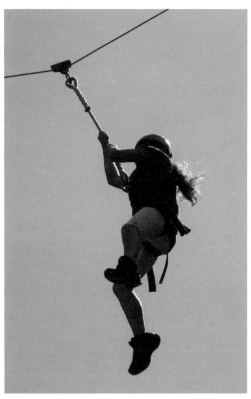

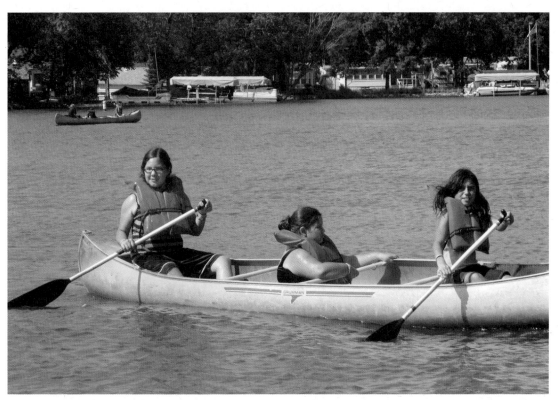

When?

Sunday, July 31 – Friday, August 5, 2011. Contact us or our website for dates of future years.

Where?

Lutherdale Camp, Elkhorn, Wisconsin

How do I learn more?

Contact the Alzheimer's & Dementia Alliance of Wisconsin, or *forMemory*, Inc.

How do I help?

Ask for a speaker to address your civic, community, or congregational group. Consider tax-deductible contributions to the scholarship fund to insure no youth are left out.

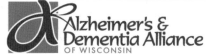

Alzheimer's & Dementia Alliance
OF WISCONSIN

formerly the Alzheimer's Association South Central Wisconsin Chapter

517 N. Segoe Rd. Suite 301, Madison, WI 53705
608-232-3400   toll free: 888-308-6251
www.alzwisc.org

forMemory, Inc.
821 W. Browning Street, Appleton, WI 54914
920-734-9638   www.forMemory.org

LUTHERDALE
N7891 US Hwy 12, Elkhorn, WI 53121
262-742-2352   www.Lutherdale.org

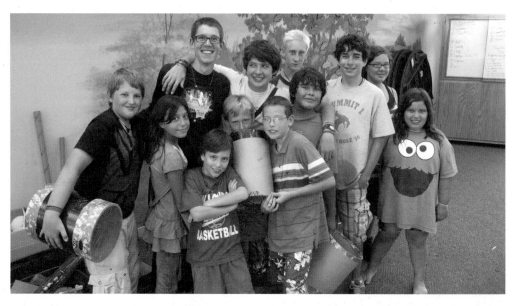

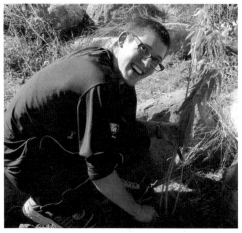

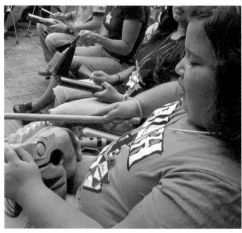

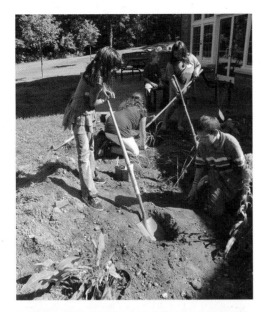

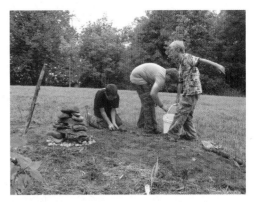

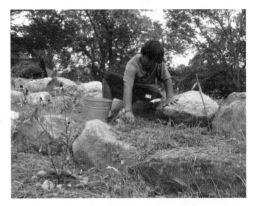

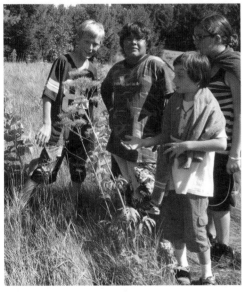

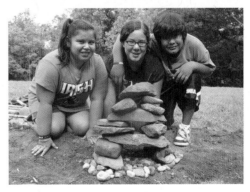

The 2010 Time for Us camp started a new emphasis on locally grown produce and on restoring nature. Activities included tasting healthy foods and spices, learning about native Queen of the Prairie already blooming on the grounds, and planting wetland prairie plants such as marsh milkweed. In order to preserve soil and water the youth planted a rain garden near their housing. They learned more about each plant as they painted markers. Finally they moved last year's Inukshuk (stone statue that marks a special place) to their rain garden. All of us celebrated the beat of nature through drums we created. Youth looked up to medical student volunteer, Josh Shapiro (facing page, bottom left), as he answered questions about brain health.

The most important lessons were strategies shared spontaneously youth to youth. A 16 year old who lives with a father with advanced Alzheimer's explained that when his repeating of the same question gets to her, she goes outside and lets off steam by yelling. This taught all of us something about taking care of ourselves in challenging situations.

Documentary and Speakers Bureau

The primary project of *forMemory* is reaching out to the public with hope for the future. Through the use of a documentary, curriculum, DVDs, resource materials and a speakers bureau, *forMemory* provides first-hand training on living well with early onset cognitive changes. Congregations, civic groups, professionals, and the public learn about cognitive health in settings that do not stigmatize. They overcome fear and denial in order to take appropriate steps for wellness, wholeness and healing. Our training instills hope and empowers broader participation and advocacy for early intervention, prevention efforts, environmental health, and healing of symptoms.

The Hope of Alzheimer's: An Advocate's Journey is a multi-media project that started by chronicling the story of activist Mary Kay Baum, a woman with early onset Alzheimer's disease, four years ago. The television production company Triangle Media Works followed Mary Kay as she advocated for people and families affected by Alzheimer's. The project includes a website, magazine articles, news stories and, eventually, a documentary and book.

"Mary Kay is one of the bravest people I've met," says Dan Smith, executive producer of Triangle Media Works. "For her to share her experience, for her to dedicate her life to early intervention, for her to use the words 'hope' and 'Alzheimer's' in the same sentence is a remarkable undertaking and we're proud to be part of it."

The project quickly expanded to include the rest of Mary Kay's family because they are integral to Mary Kay's hope. Mary Kay Baum and her sisters Chris Van Ryzin and Rosann Milius are three women who refuse to accept the diagnosis of early onset Alzheimer's or Mild Cognitive Impairment as a death sentence. The documentary has evolved even further into a broader story of *forMemory*, our Time for Us youth camp, and research into early-in-life cognitive changes.

Triangle Media Works is a television program production company based in Madison, Wisconsin. Their programs appear on Discovery, Animal Planet, National Geographic Channels International, Bravo and The Hallmark Channel.

But the project is not only a compelling documentary which will be shown on Wisconsin and Iowa Public Television in later 2011. The documentary itself involves personal and community transformation efforts. Local phone banks will be scheduled with the television showings to provide support and opportunities to viewers.

This documentary will also be available for showing in local communities in settings where discussions can follow. The discussions will include persons with early cognitive changes to tell their own story to the group assembled in the local theatre or community center. This book will be available for attendees to take home, spreading the word of hope even farther.

Through the assistance of Wheat Ridge Ministries, Wisconsin Assisted Living Association, Wisconsin Coalition of Aging Groups, and many caring living communities, *forMemory* has already developed a strong reputation for its speakers bureau.

We urge readers to consider inviting one of *forMemory*'s speaker's bureau members to speak at a local club, congregation, civic group, employee group, or assisted living home. Many times Continuing Education Units can be arranged for professional staff who attend. And regional or national gatherings benefit from a highly motivational keynote address from members of our speakers bureau.

The individuals featured in this book are living well with their cognitive changes and are happy to share their story. Contact the email address at the end of each story or call Chris at (920) 734-9638 for more contact details. Nothing seems to move an audience more than hearing directly from persons with cognitive changes who are living out their hope for a healthier world.

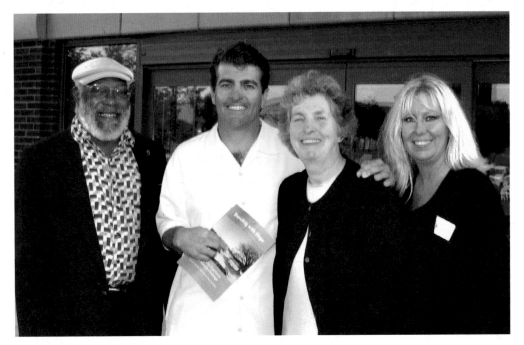

Darryl White and Mary Kay Baum spoke at Beloit Memorial Hospital on June 16, 2009. L to R Darryl White, Jonathan Moyer, Mary Kay Baum, and Kim Mason. Moyer and Mason are staff to Harbor House Assisted Living who arranged an extensive series of speaking engagements in community settings around Wisc. in 2009 and 2011. See www.myharborhouse.com.

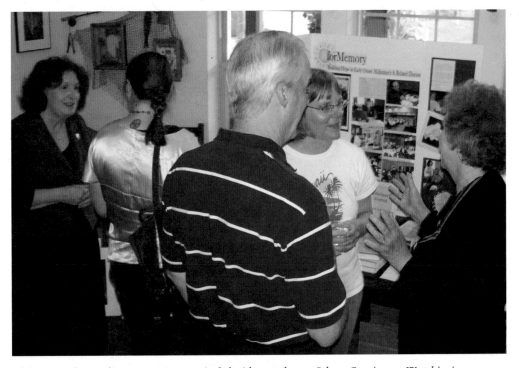

Chris Van Ryzin and Mary Kay Baum mingled with attendees at Sylvan Crossings at Westshire in Waunakee after speaking there Sept. 24, 2009 on "Living Well with Alzheimer's."

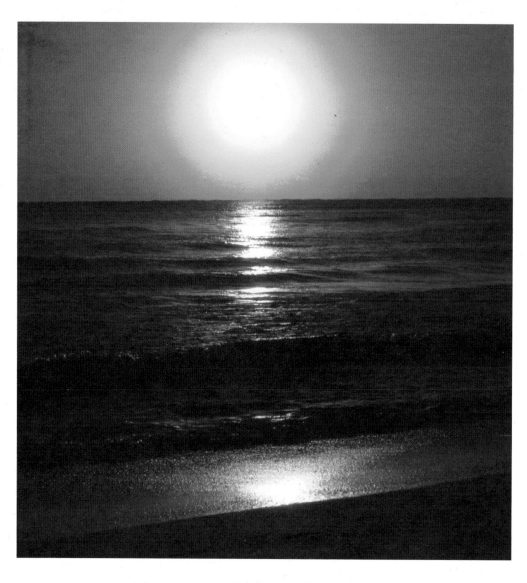

The SUN is the logo of *forMemory*
and symbolizes our hope
for healthy living.

Each sunrise reminds us
that we have another day
during which to move toward wellness
for ourselves,
our families,
our communities,
and the universe.

IV. What We Need to Know and Do

"As a physician I am concerned about giving people false hope. . . .
However, I feel strongly that if we do not tell people of all the things
that science tells us that we can do with diet, exercise, managing stress
and protecting ourselves from contaminants in the environment,
if we don't tell them all that—we are giving false hopelessness.
My fight today is against false hopelessness."

—David Servan-Schreiber, M.D., Ph.D.,
neuroscientist and survivor of brain cancer

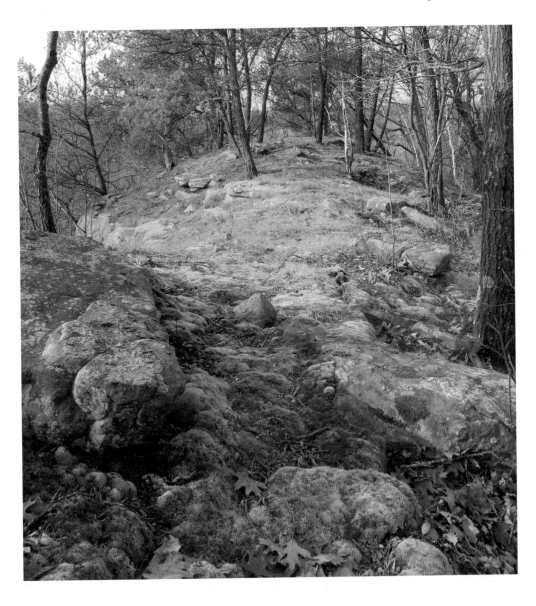

Exercise and Physical Capacity

Physical exercise may be the single most important treatment for early Alzheimer's and other dementias. One study found that those who are physically active at least twice a week in midlife had more than a 50 percent reduction in the risk of dementia type diseases in later life. People who exercise regularly reduce levels of oxidative stress and inflammatory burden. Exercise encourages new brain cells to form and enables new brain cell connections. Each of the three types of exercise: aerobic, weight training, and stretching are important because each enhances brain function differently.

But it is those with undiagnosed Alzheimer's who are often the least able to exercise. Physical frailty is probably a very early non-cognitive manifestation of Alzheimer's. This should come as no surprise. Studies have shown that motor function, grip strength, and gait speed predict Alzheimer's. Alzheimer's may impair neural systems that handle the planning and monitoring of even simple movements. Even walking is a cognitive task. Grip strength and body mass index are significantly linked to Alzheimer's brain changes, with gait changes showing a trend for an association with Alzheimer's.

How do we get out of this Catch-22? Physicians need to intervene with treatment strategies for anyone who is experiencing falling, lack of coordination, or simply a reduced desire to engage in previously preferred physical activities. Such persons may be feeling the effects of early Alzheimer's.

Many of us who are diagnosed with Alzheimer's or a related illness may be avoiding the exercise regimes we used to like because we now feel uncertain of ourselves physically. We may even have an unconscious fear of falling. Shaming us or putting more guilt

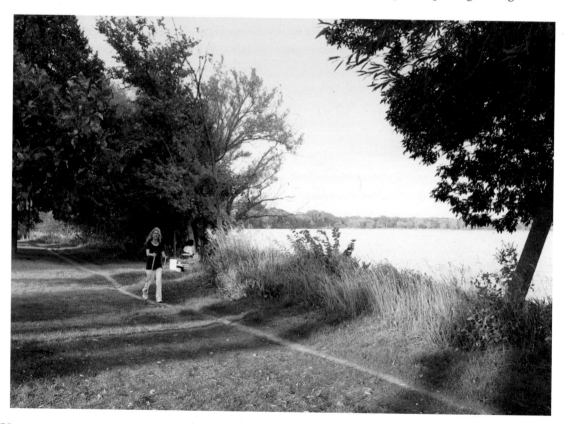

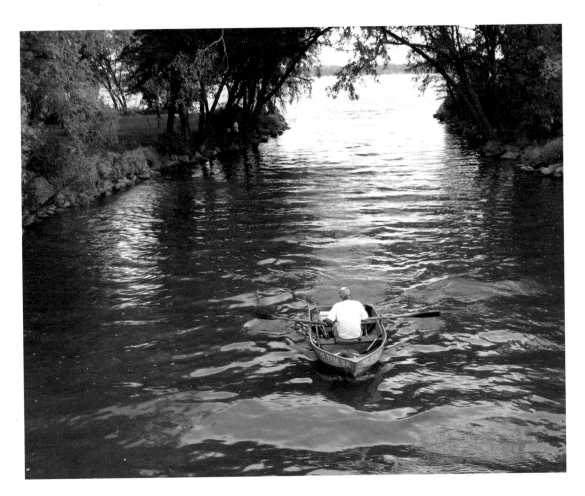

on us than we already feel will not help. We need help to address what is keeping us from physical exercise.

Dr. Valentin Bragin, M.D. Ph.D. teaches simple hand movements that can be done while sitting to improve physical coordination and activate the brain. He noticed that many of us with early-onset dementias have problems performing functions that require simultaneous use of fingers on both hands. His light, repetitive hand exercises help overall coordination and concentration. Then physical exercise may become easier.

Some of us are able to restart an exercise regime with a modified yoga class. For some, CranioSacral Therapy gives us new energy and capacity. Others have found that doing physical therapy exercises, especially for balance, is what we need to continue exercising.

What a relief! We hadn't been lazy. We just need extra help to stay active and to enjoy walking and physical exercise again.

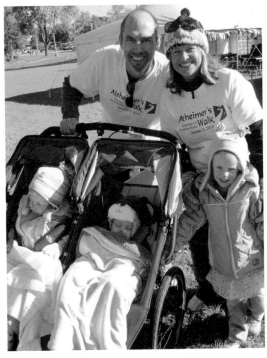

Enhancing Health for Generations

Our health is dictated not only by our genetic makeup, but also by factors that regulate the expression of proteins from our genetic code (epigenetics). Age, diet and environmental exposures affect how our genes are expressed, turning them on or off with dramatic consequences for our health. Evidence suggests that some epigenetic changes are heritable from one generation to the next. So dietary and environmental factors that alter gene expression in one individual may influence gene expression in his/her descendants. Thus, our health can be deeply connected to earlier stages of life and the world around us.

Environmental exposures, including what we eat, drink, and breathe together with stress can affect our health and therefore the progression and prevention of memory-related diseases.

Much research is now being performed in this new area that will tell us what factors influence our genes and the proteins produced by these genes. We all want to know what could help or hinder us and possibly our children. We are advocating for more definitive scientific data about the aging process, nutrition, nurturing and environment that might help turn off our troublesome genes and/or turn on our helpful ones.

Efforts have been made to pull together what data exists on how our environment and diet affect health. On October 23, 2008, "Environmental Threats to Healthy Aging" was published by Greater Boston Physicians for Social Responsibility and the Science and Environmental Health Network. This analysis of recent studies on the effects of environment is available in its entirety at www.agehealthy.org. The analysis

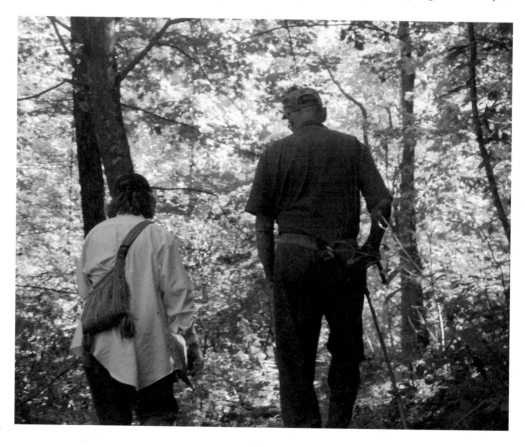

underscores that there is an entire web of biological, social, economic, and cultural factors that influences our health. The presence of certain genes may increase the risks of these diseases, but the diseases are clearly affected by environmental factors. Mostly we learn that we need much more scientific research on enhancing health for generations.

DIETARY CONSIDERATIONS

Those of us in *forMemory* concur that we feel better when we have better nutrition. We just feel better eating protein, whole grains, oats, beans, sweet potatoes, berries, cherries, apples and pears. We especially appreciate organic foods that are local and fresh. We avoid highly processed foods that are calorie-rich and nutrient-lacking. We know that in the general public there is an increased use of refined sugars, artificial sweeteners and corn syrup. But products that may be safe for the general public may cause problems for those of us who already have neurological conditions.

Combinations

Many studies have focused on a single nutrient and not gotten any significant results. There are almost no studies on the combined effects of various nutrients and broad dietary patterns. We feel this is where research is really needed . . . on combinations of healthy foods. In our own lives, just adding one "good" dietary habit (such as more cabbage family vegetables) doesn't seem to help us much. But we do find that adopting a holistic approach to diet, lifestyle, and exercise really does make us feel better.

Other Diet Traditions

We have heard a lot about the Mediterranean lifestyle which includes fresh fruit and vegetables, legumes, whole grains, fish, nuts, and olive oil. The typical Japanese diet is another to consider closely. Over the long term, these sustainable ways of eating may reduce risks associated with many neurological diseases.

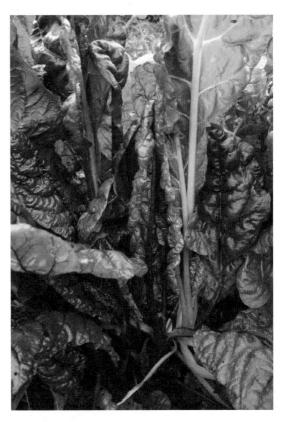

Fruits and Vegetables

High intake of fruits and vegetables is associated with decreased risks of cognitive decline. This is mostly supported by studies in animals. The benefits of fruits and vegetables are thought to be due to various antioxidant and bioactive components. Among vegetables, leafy greens, kale, spinach, onions, garlic, cabbage family (including broccoli) and beets may be especially helpful.

Flavonoids

French studies, with over 1,300 participants, showed intake of flavonoids (citrus fruit, berries, ginkgo biloba, onions, parsley, and resveratrol, which is found in white and green tea, red wine, and very dark chocolate), was associated with improved cognition in humans. At five years, the adjusted relative risk of dementia was cut approximately in half for those in the highest two thirds of flavonoid intake compared to the lowest. At 10 years, those in the lowest quartile of flavonoid intake had lost an average of

53

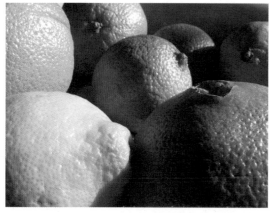

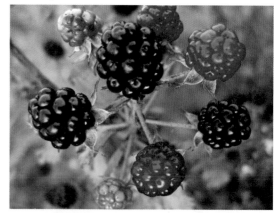

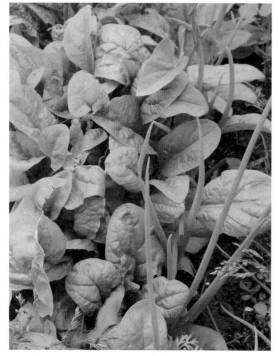

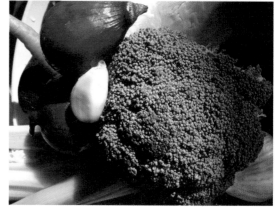

2.1 points on the Mini-Mental State Exam, compared with a loss of only 1.2 points among those in the highest quartile of flavonoid intake. Again more research is needed to confirm these results.

Plant Polyphenols

These are a kind of natural antioxidant thought to be responsible for some health benefits of fruits and vegetables. The polyphenol curcumin, which is contained in the spice turmeric, reduced levels of amyloid and plaque burden. Likewise blueberry extracts are shown to prevent and even improve memory performance and increase neurogenesis. Polyphenols may also act as scavengers of free radicals.

Folate

Higher dietary folate intake seems associated with reduced risk of developing Alzheimer's disease. Those in the highest quartile

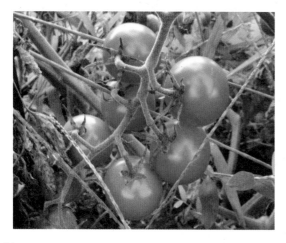

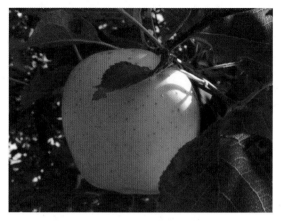

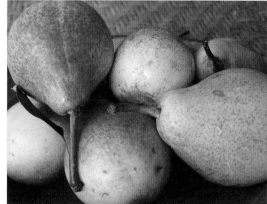

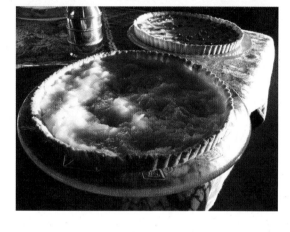

of folate intake showed half the risk of developing Alzheimer's disease compared to the lowest quartile. Rich sources of folate include legumes (lentils, chick peas), green leafy vegetables (spinach, turnip greens, lettuces), and sunflower seeds.

Spices

Spices like turmeric, rosemary, ginger, oregano, thyme, mint, cinnamon and basil are easy to add to foods and often provide health benefits.

Omega-3 and Omega-6

Both omega-3 and omega-6 are essential fatty acids important to normal health when ingested in appropriate amounts. Unfortunately, the modern American diet contains excessive amounts of omega-6's relative to omega-3's. Omega-6's appear to promote inflammation. The use of omega-6 oils, that is not offset by use of omega-3-rich oils or fish oil, more than doubles the risk of dementia. And in an animal study, restoring omega-3's alone (without reducing high intake of omega-6 fatty acids) did not reverse an observed learning impairment. Conversely, omega-3's reduce inflammation and clotting. One study reported that people with the highest blood levels of omega-3's are about half as likely to develop dementia as those with lower levels of omega-3's. A Minneapolis study of over 2,200 people aged 50–60 years found that omega-3 intake was associated with less decline in verbal fluency. Omega-3 fatty acids are found in deep yellow and dark green vegetables, walnuts, seaweed, flax seed, and foods from animals who take in green plants or algae in their food chains—including fish and animals fed on green pasture. Typically these foods have a short shelf life. Adding flax to products (like peanut butter) increases their omega-3's. Omega-6 fatty acids are found in most grains and are concentrated in corn, soy, safflower, peanut and other common vegetable oils and their products (especially fast foods). Since omega-3's are in green plants, the replacement of our grazing farms with grain-feeding factory farms has diminished the omega-3 content of dairy, beef, chicken, eggs and other animal products. Now these products typically contain increased levels of omega-6's and saturated fat (see below). To get a better balance into our diets, we need to reduce omega-6 intake and increase omega-3's. Most *forMemory* people take purified fish oil capsules daily.

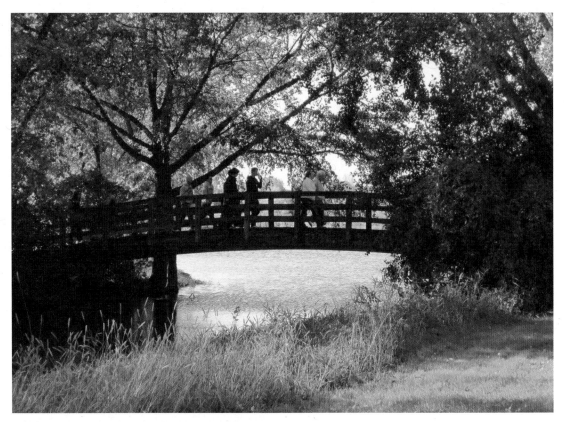

markers of inflammation. Today's diet of trans and saturated fats and high levels of omega-6's likely contributes to cognitive decline and other diseases. Higher intake of saturated fats may increase the risk of dementia by two to three times. Saturated fats are increased in fatty meats from confined, grain-fed animals, which provide most animal-based foods in the U.S. Baked goods and margarine usually contain saturated fat.

Melatonin

The supplement melatonin appears to improve memory and learning. Melatonin levels normally decline with age, but the reduction is worse in people with Alzheimer's, even in their earliest stages. A therapeutic trial in Alzheimer's patients concluded that melatonin supplements can help stabilize cognitive decline. This makes sense because inexpensive melatonin is often taken to improve sleep patterns. Sleeplessness is one of the most common problems of persons with Alzheimer's as it leads to fatigue. Avoiding

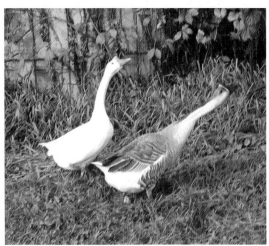

Saturated Fats

Between 1950 and 1999 annual per-person consumption of fats and oils increased by 78 percent. Dramatic increases in fried foods in the fast-food industry helped raise fat consumption. Trans fats have not only lowered levels of good cholesterol and raised bad cholesterol, but they also sharply increased over-the-counter "PM" pain relievers for sleeplessness is a good idea because their regular use may reduce speed in processing.

ENVIRONMENTAL EXPOSURES

Virtually all people and wildlife are regularly exposed to industrial chemicals that in earlier human history did not exist. Many of these synthetic chemicals have never been tested for their effects on the brain, and the synergistic effects of these chemicals is largely unexplored.

Although definitive evidence awaits further research, below is a list of chemicals that have been implicated in neurological disease.

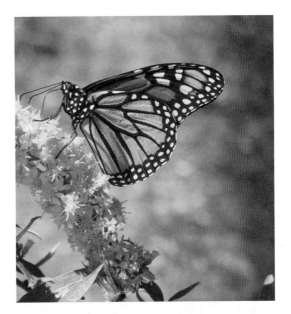

Air Pollution

Air quality alerts remind us that air pollution is harmful to humans. Living in a highly polluted city may be harder on the brain than living in clean air cities. A dietary imbalance of omega-6's to omega-3's discussed above may further exacerbate air pollution's association with cognitive impairments.

Pesticides

Over 18,000 pesticides are licensed in the USA and over two billion pounds of pesticides are applied annually to crops, homes, schools, parks, and forests, creating potential for pervasive human exposure. For those who already have memory challenges, chronic low dose exposure to a number of pesticides—primarily in the work setting—might further impair memory and attention. In one university clinic, 21 percent of 1,000 patients presenting for cognitive disorders likely had toxic exposure. Those of us with early-onset memory challenges who met each other in *forMemory* noticed that many of us lived for a long time in an environment where multiple pesticides were used. This is now a question being asked in some Alzheimer's registries in order to collect data on pesticide impact. Environmental exposure seems to lower the age at which cognitive

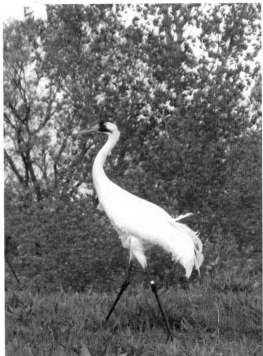

decline begins by the same degree as if carrying two copies of ApoE4, the most common mutation responsible for Alzheimer's.

Lead

Environmental lead exposure is linked to an increased risk of cognitive impairment in children. It is likely that exposures in infancy and childhood may increase the risk of memory disease decades later.

Aluminum

Dietary exposure to aluminum salts is nearly universal in the developed world. They are commonly added to commercially prepared foods and beverages. They can be used to clarify drinking water, make salt free-pouring, color foods, and make baked goods rise. The European Food Safety Authority and the Joint Food and Agriculture/WHO Expert Committee on Food Additives recently lowered their recommended safe upper limit for aluminum. Their new limit is seven times more protective than the US recommended limit. Many Americans ingest more than WHO's stringent limit through additives in processed foods and beverages. Some bak-ing powder, pancake and waffle mixes, and ready-to-eat frozen pancakes contain the most aluminum of foods tested. Consuming high-aluminum foods on a daily basis may reach exposures that increase memory loss. We purchase only baking powder that is labeled "Aluminum-Free."

Bisphenol A

BPA is a component of polycarbonate plastic bottles and some food can liners. Exposure to BPA is common because of leaching from plastic baby bottles, water bottles and other products. It remains controversial as to whether BPA is toxic, but the longer a liquid sits in such a container, the hotter the conditions, or the older the container, then the higher the risk of leaching. BPA is found in many plastic bottles marked #07 or #03-PVC.

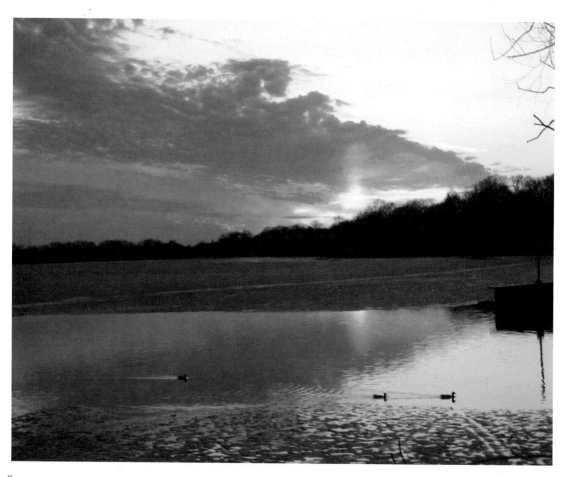

NATURE

A growing body of scientific evidence indicates that nature can help heal people's minds and bodies. There are benefits of both looking at nature and being in nature. Views of nature can speed healing, reduce need for pain medications, and improve mood. Healing gardens are therapeutic. Looking at plants, trees and animals is good for mental and emotional health, and can even sustain attention. Interacting with nature is a health tonic. Gardening reduces stress. Wilderness experiences are beneficial for cognitive disabilities. Jogging in the green outdoors seems to provide greater positive feelings than the same activity in a gym. Horticultural therapy can be a beneficial influence on everything from heart disease to dementia. The growing body of evidence suggests that people benefit so much physically and mentally from contact with nature that it should be considered a strategy for improved public health.

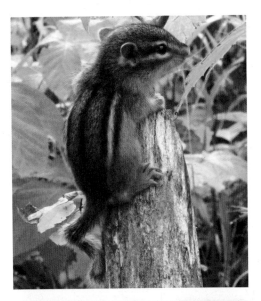

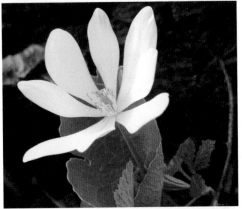

ENVIRONMENTAL STEPS THAT COULD REDUCE AGE-RELATED COGNITIVE DECLINE

Risks for Alzheimer's and related dementias can be reduced through good public policy.

- Encouraging localized, diversified and sustainable food production would enhance access to healthy food, cut down on its harmful content, decrease the environmental impacts of agriculture, and strengthen local economies. Local foods could reduce reliance on pesticides and minimize the use of fossil fuels for long distance transport. This would further reduce pollution and greenhouse gas emissions.

- Energy policies that reduce toxic emissions, promote conservation and efficiency, and curtail dependence on fossil fuels will also encourage physical activity. Clean energy reduces harmful

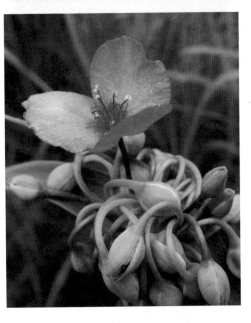

chemical exposures of producing, transporting and using fossil fuels. Developing energy-efficient transit systems that interface with bike paths and sidewalk networks saves energy while minimizing air pollution and combating obesity. Of course living closer to one's work site is best of all.

- Reducing use of toxic substances in the home, workplace, and community through regulatory reform, "safer substitute" programs, and green product design can reduce toxic exposures, reduce ecosystem contamination, and create new jobs.

- Reducing socioeconomic disparities and making certain that all people have access to affordable health care, primary prevention and a decent environment will reduce chronic disease burdens on society.

- Increasing awareness of the link between head injuries at any age and cognitive decline.

Integrative Medicine

Integrative medicine incorporates complementary techniques such as nutraceuticals, stress reduction, acupuncture, massage, and yoga. Physical, mental, emotional, social, and spiritual paths are addressed to find the most effective and least invasive ways to optimize health. Acupuncture is most commonly used to treat chronic pain, stress, anxiety, fatigue, insomnia, and depression, all of which if reduced can positively impact dementia and Alzheimer's disease.

A simple ancient yoga practice may stimulate neuro-pathways in the brain. Stand with feet forward about shoulder width apart, grab the right earlobe with thumb and finger of the left hand. Cross the right arm over the left and grab the left earlobe with the right hand. Then squat down as fully as you can while breathing in. Then stand back up breathing out. Repeat this motion working up to three minutes a day. Yale neurobiologist Eugenius Ang, Jr., Ph.D., said,

"Holding the left ear activates the right brain while holding the right ear activates the left brain." He said EEG readings in his study of the practice showed right and left hemispheres of the brain had become more synchronized

Reducing Toxins

Some researchers call us "canaries in the mine." This is because we provide a warning call when there are toxins in the environment. Because Alzheimer's compromises our blood/brain barriers we are much more affected by harmful substances.

Many times foods are advertised as healthy, but may not be healthy for some of us.

We are NOT content to remain "canaries in the mine." We want to be more like the bald eagle. The eagle was once endangered by pesticides like DDT. It was, in part, concern for the eagle that resulted in the regulation of pesticides. We, too, want to help effect change to benefit ourselves and our ecosystems.

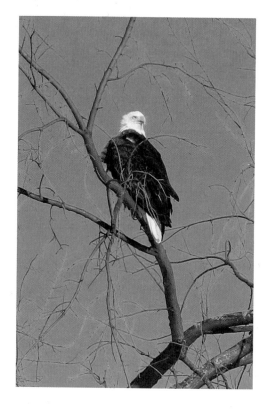

Finding Out If I Might Have Alzheimer's: A Long Process

"I worry about my forgetfulness. Could I have Alzheimer's? What can I do to find out?" are questions often asked of us. There are many different causes for cognitive changes. Early intervention may not only find other treatable causes but also extend quality of life. People are affected in differing ways and no one has all the following signs of concern. The following steps may help you obtain early and effective help.

Ask yourself the following, knowing there may be many other explanations for these changes:

1. Am I now avoiding social or physical activities that I used to enjoy . . . especially if they are in the evening?

2. Am I less coordinated now? Am I falling, running into objects, or dropping things more than my old self?

3. Do I have disturbed or changed sleep patterns? Am I routinely more tired in the morning than before?

4. Am I getting sad, anxious, upset, angry, startled, or fearful more often than before?

5. Am I more defensive about criticism, more irritable, or less patient with others than before?

6. Am I less able to stay on task at work or in household roles?

7. Are supervisors or peers expressing concerns about my work performance?

8. Is it harder and taking me longer to do tasks that I used to do easily without much thought?

9. Do I have trouble keeping track of time and get so absorbed in things that I forget my other duties?

10. Do I have more trouble finding my words now? Do I lose my train of thought more often?

11. Is it harder to pay attention, especially if there is noise or commotion around me?

12. Am I more worn out by conversation and group activity than before?

13. Am I more tired and in pain from physical activities like walking?

14. Am I having a harder time remembering details from long ago?

15. Do I have more trouble remembering recent things like where I parked or put my keys?

16. Is it harder to learn a new activity now than it used to be to learn a new activity years ago?

17. Is it harder to make decisions, multitask, lead groups, or give instructions now?

18. Am I feeling overwhelmed or overloaded more than I used to?

19. Do I compensate through more reminders to myself or working longer hours?

20. Am I bothered by heat or coldness, by odors or scents, by cleaning supplies or food additives?

21. Am I getting new, more, or worse headache, tremor, dizziness, bright light aura, pain, gazing off, or weakness?

22. In summary, do I notice any subtle physical, mental, vocational, emotional or social changes in myself?

To help physicians determine the source of these changes, did some appear after a fall, operation, illness, stroke, concussion, greater stress, menopause, or medication change? Which ones? Finally, write down any low or high blood pressure, low or high cholesterol, and any blood sugar issues.

- Now share your answers with loved one(s). Sincerely ask for feedback on any changes they notice.

- Organize any of these concerns in writing, noting dates and frequency.

- Write a personal and family history of dementia, neurological, or chronic conditions like diabetes, ALS, substance abuse or mental illness.

- Write down the times you may have experienced toxic contamination (i.e. lead, pesticides, war service.

- Before proceeding, consider obtaining the best health insurance, public benefits, disability insurance and long-term care insurance that you still can.

- If you have a trusted family physician, start with an appointment there. Be aware that not every doctor understands memory challenges or handles subtle early signs well. A second opinion may be needed.

- Go to the appointment with a loved one(s). Consider bringing an additional, note-taking advocate.

- Give one copy of your concerns to the doctor, one to your note-taker, and keep one in front of you.

- Informed physicians will speak to you directly. They will ask loved ones about their impressions and may order blood tests. The physician may give a mini-mental exam or other short screening device, even knowing these tools are not sensitive to early changes. They will make sure you are not dehydrated. They may work with you on depression issues, knowing Alzheimer's also brings its own chemical depression.

- A referral to a neurologist or memory clinic shows your physician understands his/her limitations. Ideally you will maintain your primary care physician for overall health issues and have him/her receive reports from any specialists. But if your physician dismisses all your concerns out of hand, you need to locate a physician or neurologist who listens. Even some neurologists specialize elsewhere and do not handle cognitive issues well.

- Schedule a neuropsychological assessment through a neurologist, memory clinic, or veterans or university hospital. These often last two to three hours. The earlier you have a neuropsychological, the more helpful it will be as a baseline for the future.

- Afterwards a psychologist will explain the assessment results or send them to your doctor. Ask for a written copy. It compares you to average persons at your age and years of education. It may show weak areas and strengths. An exam two years later may show if there is cognitive decline. Often even a tentative diagnosis is not given until a decline is seen among your "neuropsychs." How you do on a particular "neuropsych" may depend on the time of day and how you are feeling that day.

- You might be referred for an MRI, other scans, and/or EEG. Ask to keep a copy at time of scan.

- Now comes the most unpredictable time in your diagnosis process. Some physicians will order just one "neuropsych," attach the label Alzheimer's disease without ruling out other possibilities, and quickly prescribe a well-known Alzheimer's drug. Others seem to attribute everything to depression and ignore family history and Parkisonian or seizure symptoms. Still others will not use the term Alzheimer's until an autopsy after death and may merely annually monitor gradual decline into advanced dementia. A second opinion may be helpful.

- We in *forMemory* advocate for early interventions to reduce our symptoms. We seek ways including nutrition and life style changes to improve quality of life and manage our own unique set of symptoms. We may coordinate with our neurologist both Western medicine and integrative alternatives to help reduce tremor and sleep disturbance.

- We advocate for help such as balance physical therapy and specific medications for pain and falling. All doctors recognize that regular physical activity is essential for Alzheimer's patients. But many forget that it is hard to exercise when there is pain and fear of falling. Medical intervention is required in these cases. Some neurologists are now prescribing the Selegiline Patch for those with Parkinsonian-type symptoms because it reduces these symptoms, while it manages chemical depression and is neuro-protective.

- Neurologists who follow current research know that seizure activity may be causing cognitive damage well before seizures are clinically apparent. The EEG's they routinely order indicate whether there is seizure activity that would warrant medication.

If there is a showing of cognitive decline consider joining *forMemory*'s database at www.formemorydatabase.org.

Consider joining a registry or clinical trial if you are eligible. But remember these trials are for research and you might not get any results for your use. While in a study you still need your own neurologist and treatment plan.

Regardless of your neurological status, consider arranging for a Brain Bank to autopsy your brain upon your death to help research. This can be an important gift for your children, future generations, and all communities.

If you have concerns about others, you might suggest that getting a neuropsychological assessment is good for a baseline.

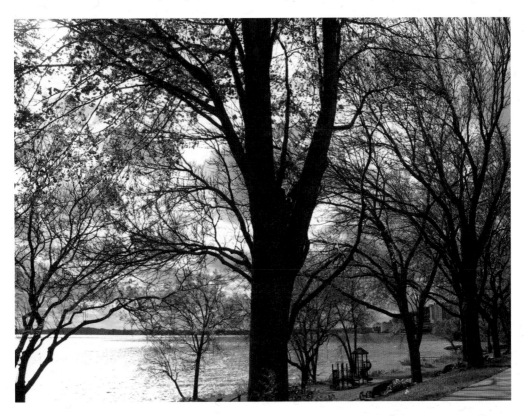

Online, Print and Other Resources

Alzheimer's Averted: A Path to Survival is authored by *forMemory*'s very own Chris Baum Van Ryzin (read about Chris at page 16). Self-published as a hard cover book in 2004, a 2010 soft cover edition is now available for $18 at *forMemory* events, through Elemental Basic Publishing, www.alzheimersaverted .com or by calling Chris at (920) 734-9638. "Avert" is defined as to see coming, to ward off, avoid, prevent. These were the goals of Chris when in 1989 at the early age of 41 she experienced symptoms similar to her mother's (later autopsy confirmed early onset Alzheimer's). Chris sought cross-generational care from the neurologist who treated her mother. The book is written in the form of the diary her neurologist requested her to keep, with her added research and first hand knowledge, complemented by the touching poetry written to "help find my words." *Alzheimer's Averted* shares the path Chris took to not only slow the progression but to also re-

learn to live using a whole mind, body, spirit approach to healing. She tells her story so others will benefit, bringing hope, planting seeds of involvement, and adding the word "survivor" to cognitive decline. Many persons with early-in-life cognitive changes call her story their "Alzheimer's Bible."

Beyond Alzheimer's: How to Avoid the Modern Epidemic of Dementia by Scott D. Mendelson, M.D., Ph.D., a psychiatrist with 15 years of neuroscience research who consults at an Oregon veterans hospital, was published in Sept. 2009 by M. Evans & Company. This $19 hardcover book gives the public a comprehensive, positive and balanced view of prevention strategies. Dr. Mendelson explains research on nutraceuticals such as ashwagandha, turmeric, garlic, melatonin, and fish oil. He urges us to stop metabolic syndrome, embrace food as medicine, maintain ideal weight, exercise, get quality sleep,

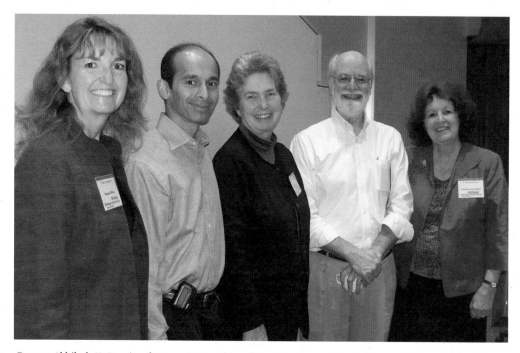

Doctors Abhilash K. Desai and George T. Grossberg of the Department of Psychiatry and Human Behavior, Saint Louis University Health Science Center meet frequently with members of forMemory and share materials.

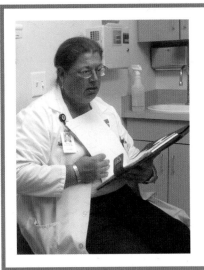

Neurologist **Janelle Cooper, M.D.,** director of the Memory Center at Gundersen Lutheran Neurosciences in LaCrosse, Wisconsin, was honored with the Outstanding Physician Award at the 2010 Wisconsin State Alzheimer's conference in recognition of her work on behalf of patients with Alzheimer's disease and related memory disorders. Dr. Cooper is a board-certified neurologist with a subspecialty in behavioral neurology and an emphasis and research interest in memory loss. Her current research focus is on the role of vitamins B5 and B7 in the development of memory loss.

treat sleep apnea, avoid environmental toxins (including radon and air pollution), treat depression (including with diet), exercise our mind, and stay socially active. He believes that while some genes increase risk, dementia results mostly from the acquisition of various risk factors throughout life. Dr. Mendelson is a frequent guest on public radio and The Huffington Post, commenting on dementia risks to our war veterans and to athletes with repeated head impact. He calls for holistic, comprehensive public policy changes to provide treatment for risk factors and to reduce toxin exposure. On Wisconsin Public Radio Mendelson affirmed that the selegiline patch is a good neuroprotective antioxidant that is an MAO inhibiting antidepressant and reduces Parkinsonian symptoms as it helps with the dopamine.

Healthy Brain Aging: Evidence Based Methods to Preserve Brain Function and Prevent Dementia was compiled by Psychiatrist Dr. Abhilash Desai for the Feb. 2010 Clinics in Geriatric Medicine. Dr. Desai is a scientific advisor to *forMemory* and practiced in Appleton, Wisconsin and St. Louis, Missouri. He says, "I am optimistic that these data will contribute to the development of interventions that generate action in local communities and eventually result in improved public health. This is . . . an invitation to every clinician, individual, and family to make healthy brain aging a priority."

To maximize cardiovascular and brain health, Dr. Desai recommends people become FEISTY, an acronym for his program of lifestyle habits.

F = Food: Recent studies suggest that a Mediterranean diet, with lots of fruits, vegetables, fish and olive oil, can reduce the risk of cognitive decline.

E = Exercise: Daily aerobic exercise is best for the brain, although any regular exercise can help.

I = Intellect: Taking on new and intellectually challenging activities throughout life keeps the brain active and builds new connections in the brain. This can be anything that challenges the mind, from learning a new language to starting a part-time job.

S = Sleep: Get a good night's sleep to ensure brain health, and treat conditions such as sleep apnea.

T = Treatment: It's important to treat many other health conditions, like high blood pressure or high cholesterol levels, to help reduce the risks of Alzheimer's disease.

Y = Yes: Say "yes" to opportunities in your life, from going to lunch with friends to joining a reading group.

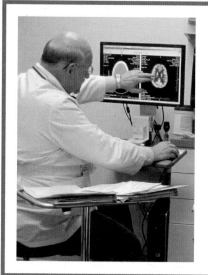

Benjamin Rix Brooks, M.D., is the Medical Director of the Carolinas Neuromuscular/ALS–MDA Center in the Department of Neurology at Carolinas Medical Center and is Professor of Neurology in this facility for the study and treatment of degenerative neuromuscular diseases. He also specializes in neurotoxic disorders (diseases of environmental origin) and has a research interest in orphan diseases which impact few patients and therefore do not attract much attention or research. Since research on orphans has been neglected, information can be scarce as well. These diseases may be abandoned, or "orphaned," because they provide little financial incentive for the private sector to make and market new medications to treat or prevent them. Most orphan diseases have a genetic component and are chronic.

Neurology Now: Healthy Living for Patients & Their Families is an official publication of the American Academy of Neurology. This informative, yet easy to read, bimonthly magazine is available at no cost to individuals with a neurological disorder, their families and caregivers. For free home delivery call 1-800-422-2681 or visit www.neurologynow.com.

The Thousand Mile Stare: One Family's Journey through the Science and Struggle of Alzheimer's is the true 30 year story of one family's discovery that it carries a gene for early onset Alzheimer's. Written by Gary Reiswig, a cousin of Chuck Jackson (see page 23), about their mutual extended family, it was published in Feb. 2010 by Nicholas Brealey Publishing. The Foreword is by renowned scientist Dr. Thomas Bird. The 240 page book lists for $22 through most book sources. Visit the author's blog, "The Thousand Mile Stare: Thinking About Alzheimer's: Yesterday, Today, Tomorrow" at http://thethousandmilestare.blogspot.com. The book is considered a "must-read" for scientists and for those with cognitive changes early in life. One reader wrote, "Gary has given me a face, as he has to his family by writing this book. I like to believe that Gary's cousin Chuck and I are LIVING with Alzheimer's not dying from it. This book keeps our fires alive. . . ."

forMemory, Inc.   www.formemory.org
The official site of *forMemory*, a network for those affected directly or indirectly by symptoms of cognitive changes that began before the age of 65 years. We advocate for better health systems, community connectedness, and a toxic-free planet. We have a passion to improve the quality of life for ourselves, our children, and future generations worldwide. Activities include research collaboration on database, camp for affected youth, peer support, education and outreach.

Alzheimer's & Dementia Alliance of Wisconsin   www.alzwisc.org
The Alzheimer's & Dementia Alliance of Wisconsin provides services to improve the quality of life for all those affected by cognitive challenges from preclinical to end-of-life stages. Emphasis is on guidance, education, support and advocacy.

Contact the Madison office at 608.232.3400 or toll-free 888.308.6251, or email support@alzwisc.org. Outreach offices include Lancaster and Portage in Southern Wisconsin.

The Hope of Alzheimer's: An Advocate's Journey is a documentary film in process about Mary Kay Baum and her sisters Chris Van Ryzin and Rosann Baum Milius—three women who refuse to accept the diagnosis of early onset Alzheimer's or of Mild Cognitive Impairment as a death sentence. Web site www.hopeofalzheimers.com gives video clips from the film, samples of Mary Kay's photos, and links to related sites.

The Tangled Neuron
www.tangledneuron.info
Mona Johnson helped set up our first *for-Memory* database. Her own website and weekly emailed articles are an excellent resource for laypersons wanting to understand today's research on memory, dementia and Alzheimer's.

Alzheimer's Daily News www.alznews.org
Mark and Ellen Warner's *Alzheimer's Daily News* provides daily subscription to excellent summaries of the latest research on Alzheimer's and related neurological diseases. They provide links to the research itself.

Dementia USA www.dementiausa.com
Information on Alzheimer's disease, dementia, memory loss, problems, and more. Includes symptoms, prevention, care giving, and treatment information.

Journal of Alzheimer's Disease
www.j-alz.com
An international multidisciplinary journal with a mission to facilitate progress in understanding the etiology, pathogenesis, epidemiology, genetics, behavior, treatment and psychology of Alzheimer's disease.

Alzheimer's Reading Room
www.alzheimersreadingroom.com
Bob DeMarco's *Alzheimer's Reading Room* stresses late stage issues because Bob cares for his 93-year-old late stage mother. But he has refreshing views and understandings that appear almost daily.

The Myth of Alzheimer's
www.themythofalzheimers.com
Peter Whitehouse, M.D., Ph.D. is author of the book of the same title. Promotes reducing stigma and making care in aging a whole community responsibility; is very critical of early testing, labeling and drug promises; does explore some very positive intergenerational approaches.

www.usagainstalzheimers.org/blog
George Vradenburg, a former media executive, and driving force behind the Alzheimer's Study Group, and his spouse Trish write this blog. Trish is author of *Surviving Grace*, a play that honors her mother who had Alzheimer's. It was produced at Kennedy Center, Off-Broadway, and internationally.

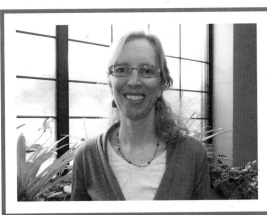

Dr. Jennifer Norden is the medical director of the Mary Kimball Anhaltzer Center for Integrative Medicine in Oshkosh, Wisconsin. She is a board-certified internist who studied integrative medicine at the Univ. of Arizona and trained in acupuncture at the Helms Medical Institute in California. She and her staff offer healing oriented therapies and classes. See www.affinityhealth.org.

www.handintheplan.org
Toward a Wisconsin State Alzheimer's Plan. Your responses to this website's surveys will be used to help draft a plan in Wisconsin to address Alzheimer's disease. Learning and Listening Sessions are being scheduled. Help develop implementable recommendations to expand current resources, make effective service and support programs widely available, enact legislative changes for systems improvements, and identify sources of funding. The state Office on Aging, the Helen Bader Foundation, and the Planning Council for Health and Human Services seek your input.

Wisc. Alzheimer's Disease Research Center:
Wisc. Comprehensive Memory Program
(WCMP) with Director Sanjay Asthana provides a systems approach to diagnosis, treatment, education, and research. It is based in the UW Hospital and VA Hospitals in Madison. To participate in a study call 608-263-2582 or toll free 1-866-636-7764. Visit www.wcmp.wisc.edu to find community education events or a Memory Clinic near you to provide detailed testing for early detection of cognitive changes.

WCMP's Brain Donor Program is a repository of tissues for research. Collecting does not interfere with funeral or viewing arrangements. It is important that persons with Alzheimer's disease, with memory concerns, or with no cognitive concerns

consider donating and registering early by calling (608) 256-1901, ext 11767.

Affiliated with WCMP, the *Wisc. Alzheimer's Institute hosts WRAP*, the largest long-term study of healthy relatives of persons with Alzheimer's disease. See www.wai.wisc.edu/research/wrap.html, or call (608) 829-3300. Recruiting African-Americans and English-speaking Hispanics/Latinos whose parent(s) developed Alzheimer's. Persons whose parents did not develop dementia are asked to become controls.

The National Academy on an Aging Society, an institute of Gerontological Society at www .policy@agingsociety.org or (202) 408-3375 provides a quarterly *Public Policy & Aging Report.* Its summer 2010 issue featured the following topics and is available for $20—$39 per year for 4 reports. "Environmental Threats to Healthy Aging—An Ecological Perspective"; "The Food Environment—Changing 50 Years of Growing an Inflammatory Diet"; "The Chemical Environment: Toxic Chemicals, Hazardous Substances, and Chronic Diseases of Aging"; "The Built Environment: Planning Healthy Communities for all Ages"; and "The Psychosocial Environment—An Intergenerational Approach." A *Public Policy & Aging* E-Newsletter is free (send an email to aging report@gmail.com with "Subscribe" in subject line).

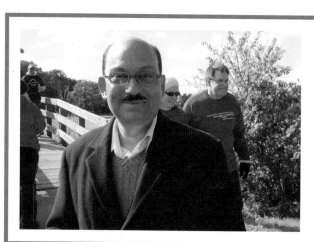

Sanjay Asthana, M.D. (Geriatrician, Internist) is Director of the Wisconsin Comprehensive Memory Program and is pictured here showing his community involvement by walking in the Alzheimer's & Dementia Alliance of Wisconsin Dane County Alzheimer's Walk.

Conclusion

"Whatever affects one directly, affects all indirectly. I can never be what I ought to be until you are what you ought to be. This is the interrelated structure of reality."
— *Dr. Martin Luther King, Jr.*

Hope Regarding Persons Already in Later Stages

We three had the privilege to accompany our mother in her last days. It was an opportunity we'll never forget and our mother continues to inform our lives. We do experience grief for the years of our mother's frustration, muteness, and pain. Both Rosann and Chris joined our father in providing direct care for Mom. We were fortunate to have a mother who accepted care graciously without a difficult personality change.

We applaud those many care providers who realize there is an opportunity in connecting with their loved one. We encourage emphasizing capabilities and empowering the loved one to continue their favorite enjoyments with adaptations. We encourage the community to stay involved.

Our hopes for persons in later stages are for the calm and supportive presence of loved ones, community-wide embracing of the entire family, regular respite opportunities, earlier hospice care, more pain relief, excellent palliative care, and widespread autopsy donations for research.

Hope for Us with Our Own Cognitive Changes

We've known for a long time that we are impacted by what we consume, what we breathe, and what we do. Now through epigenetic study we know we are also impacted by what our ancestors consumed, breathed, and did.

We have chronic health conditions and are more at risk to exposures than the average person. We pay attention when weather alerts state, "An advisory is being issued because of persistent elevated levels of fine particles in the air. These fine particles come primarily from combustion sources, such as power plants, factories and other industrial sources, vehicle exhaust, and wood burning. The Air Quality Index is currently in the orange level, which is considered unhealthy for people in sensitive groups. People in those sensitive groups include those with heart or lung disease, asthma, older adults and children. . . . Fine particle pollution deposits itself deep into the lungs and cannot easily be exhaled."

Besides avoiding substances about which there are printed health warnings, we record our own reactions like vertigo, headache, queasiness, or disorientation. One or more of us has noted physical problems from exposure to bleach, conventional fabric softeners, the chemical odor on some man-made new fabrics, chlorine or bromine treated pools, heavy gas burning traffic, coal-burning plants, wood burning smoke, newly treated potato fields, chemically fertilized soy fields, MSG, food dyes (even in medications), artificial sweeteners, cola drinks, creamer substitutes, and conventional hot dogs. We often find research underway on these very concerns.

Although independent research is not conclusive, we are wary of long-term use of cell phones close to our head and have recently stopped leaving them on in our pocket.

We are forever grateful for the impact that the patch selegiline has on our lives. Its antidepressant, anti-Parkinsonian and neuroprotective properties enable us to continue our therapeutic activities

We are often asked which supplements we use. We only use nutraceuticals under the supervision of our physician and it varies for each of us. At least two of us take purified Omega-3 fish oil, bio-identical estrodiol and prometrium hormone replacement therapy, ginko biloba, melatonin, folate in a good multi vitamin, aspirin, Prevagen apo-aequorin, gotu kola, schizandra, rhodiola, cinnamon, cranberry, garlic, vitamins A, B5, B7, C, D3, and E, Coenzyme Q10, turmeric, basil, ginger, valerian, rosemary, and lavender on a daily basis. We apply many anti-inflammatory herbs topically.

We enjoy plenty of physical, social, intellectual and creative activities. Chris saw dramatic improvements years ago as she took time for rest, nurturance, and stimulation. Mary Kay finds that the more she hikes and creates photo art in nature, the easier she finds her words. Rosann is a model for exercise, nutrition, creative arts, and meaning through caring for others. We each develop our own plan for living well with our particular cognitive changes.

While we each have some fear for our own personal futures, we experience a confidence that we are adapting, planning, and surviving well and that we are in the company of caring partners.

Our hopes for ourselves are that we continue to stay on top of any coexisting medical conditions such as seizure or stroke; that we continue our life-long learning; that if we need more care we are planning for it and will accept it graciously; that we stay connected to the community and many care partners; that we continue telling our story and advocating for necessary changes.

Hope for Others Living Now

The World Health Organization (WHO) says that advanced dementia is the fifth most common cause of death in the ageing population worldwide. The greatest increase in dementia is outside the USA. Already 58% of people with dementia live in developing countries, but by 2050 this will rise to 71%. The WHO has initiated aggressive campaigns for early awareness and interventions.

We, too, feel this urgency and add promotion of environmental protection efforts. Dementia risks might be reduced by fewer pollutants, by more physical activity, and by better nutrition. Chronic diseases typically do not have one single cause. They generally re-

sult from a whole range of things acting together. Among factors are too much intake of omega-6 fatty acids and not enough omega-3's; too much sugar and not enough vegetables; too much stress and not enough physical activity; too many hours of overtime work and too little rest; too much pollution and too little fresh air, clean water, and good soil.

Epigenetic study shows that environmental factors—from our diets to chemicals we're exposed to—accumulate over our lifetimes. The expression system of our genes is much more sensitive to environmental factors than our hard genes. Damage can occur without a gene mutation. The National Institutes of Health listed epigenetic research as one of its top priorities.

Some generations of some populations have already been affected disproportionately by toxin dumping, lead paint, and hazards in the workplace, farm field, and army field.

All people have something to contribute to the earth's healing. We need to heal and act together. If we do not come together to sustain the earth and enable it to heal, none of us will be healthy. Our wellness is tied to the wellness of the earth. Our wellbeing is tied to the wellbeing of all communities.

Our hopes for peers is that they hear messages of prevention, early intervention and treatment; that they make lifestyle and environmental changes; that they note any neurological changes in themselves; that they challenge medical practitioners to listen and to consider and monitor therapies that may reduce symptoms; that they pass on healthy epigenetic expression to their children and progeny; that they make advance directives to donate tissue to their local brain bank; and that they act for public policies that promote health and wellbeing for all communities.

We also hope that service models flourish to actualize the goals of persons with cognitive changes. Art mentors, personal physical trainers, complementary medicine practitioners, organic nutraceutical growers, public benefits specialists, pastoral care providers, family counselors, spiritual guidance directors, music therapists, movement therapists, financial and legal planners, specialized nutritionists, organic food restaurateurs, continuing education teachers, museum personnel, transportation providers, nature guides, and inter-generational activity directors would be gathered. No fee, low-fee, or barter opportunities would be available. Guidance would be provided by persons with mild cognitive changes who live in the area.

Our deepest hope is that we answer the call to listen to each other; that we join together to imagine a healthier world; and that we join with each other to create that world. Then there will be pathways of hope for all.

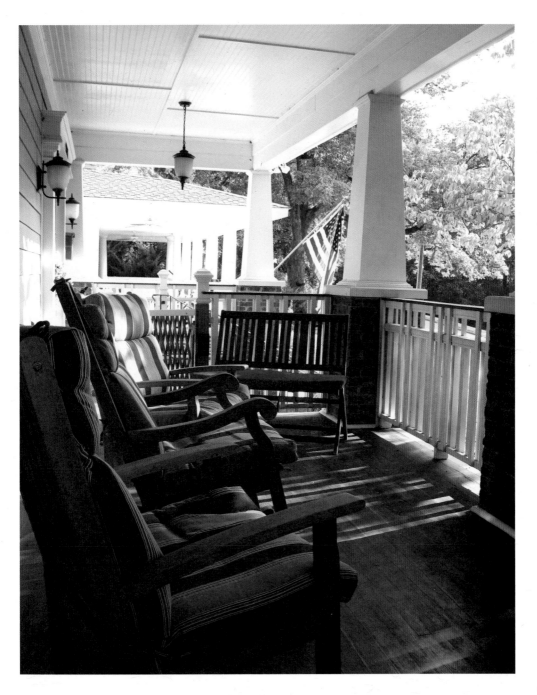

About the Co-Editors

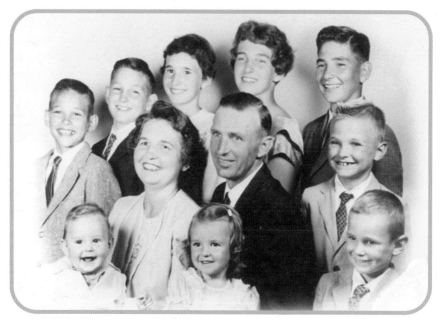

The Baum sisters with their biological family. Chris and Mary Kay are in the back row. Little sister Rosann is in front center.

Co-editors Chris Baum Van Ryzin, Mary Kay Baum, and Rosann Baum Milius are sisters who grew up on a typical Wisconsin dairy farm. They shared in the responsibilities of farm and family life with their six brothers. Early in life each developed an appreciation for the land and awe for the earth and the life within it.

Both their mother and maternal aunt experienced early-onset Alzheimer's disease coupled with vascular symptoms. Buelah, their mother, experienced neurological and sight changes, seizures, and confusion in her fifties. By two years before death in her mid-seventies, Buelah had become mute and bedridden. Although much younger, and living in the southwest, their Aunt Mabel had serious speech and spatial symptoms in her fifties and died of Alzheimer's disease in her mid-seventies also. Both mother and aunt had led lives of service and then, when it was time, each accepted care graciously, even with the fear and frustration of dementia.

The three sisters participated in their mother's neurology appointments. Each has been fortunate to be able to turn to the same research neurologist, Benjamin Rix Brooks, M.D. He had performed the autopsy for Buelah and reviewed the autopsy provided on Aunt Mabel. So Dr. Brooks has truly been a cross-generational neurologist and scientist for the sisters. Experienced with neuromuscular and motor disorders, he documents and treats the maze of related and varying issues among the sisters.

See pages 16 through 22 for the sisters' individual stories.

Contact information is as follows:

Chris Baum Van Ryzin, 821 West Browning Street, Appleton WI 54914 (920)734-9638, cbvanryzin@aol.com

Mary Kay Baum, 3819 Evans Quarry Road, Dodgeville, WI 53533 (608)935-5834, marykbaum@gmail.com

Rosann Baum Milius, 1305 Maricopa Drive, Oshkosh, WI 54904 (920)231-9237, rosann.milius@gmail.com